THOMSON DELMAR LEARNING'S
NURSING REVIEW SERIES:

Maternity and Women's Health Nursing

D1289788

THOMSON DELMAR LEARNING'S NURSING REVIEW SERIES

Maternity and Women's Health Nursing

Content taken from:
NCLEX-RN® Review

By:
Alice M. Stein EdD, RN
Retired
Senior Associate Dean for Student and Business Affairs
Drexel University
College of Nursing and Health Professions
Philadelphia, Pennsylvania

THOMSON

DELMAR LEARNING Australia   Canada   Mexico   Singapore   Spain   United Kingdom   United States

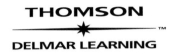

Nursing Review Series: Maternity and Women's Health Nursing

by Alice M Stein

Vice President, Health Care Business Unit:
William Brottmiller

Director of Learning Solutions:
Matthew Kane

Acquisitions Editor:
Tamara Caruso

Product Manager:
Patricia Gaworecki

Editorial Assistant:
Jenn Waters

Marketing Director:
Jennifer McAvey

Marketing Channel Manager:
Michele McTighe

Marketing Coordinator:
Danielle Pacella

Technology Director:
Laurie Davis

Technology Project Manager:
Mary Colleen Liburdi
Patricia Allen

Production Director:
Carolyn Miller

Production Manager:
Barbara Bullock

Art Director:
Robert Plante
Jack Pendleton

Content Project Manager:
Dave Buddle
Stacey Lamodi
Jessica McNavich

Production Coordinator:
Mary Ellen Cox

Library of Congress Cataloging-in-Publication Data
ISBN 1-4018-1175-2

Notice to the Reader

Publisher does not warrant or guarantee any of the products described herein or perform any independent analysis in connection with any of the product information contained herein. Publisher does not assume, and expressly disclaims, any obligation to obtain and include information other than that provided to it by the manufacturer.

The reader is expressly warned to consider and adopt all safety precautions that might be indicated by the activities described herein and to avoid all potential hazards. By following the instructions contained herein, the reader willingly assumes all risks in connection with such instructions.

The publisher makes no representations or warranties of any kind, including but not limited to, the warranties of fitness for particular purpose or merchantability, nor are any such representations implied with respect to the material set forth herein, and the publisher takes no responsibility with respect to such material. The publisher shall not be liable for any special, consequential, or exemplary damages resulting, in whole or part, from the reader's use of, or reliance upon, this material.

Contents

v

Contributors

Margaret Ahearn-Spera, RN, C, MSN
Director, Medical Patient Care Services
Danbury Hospital
Danbury, Connecticut
Assistant Clinical Professor
Yale University School of Nursing
New Haven, Connecticut

Mary Mescher Benbenek, RN, MS, CPNP, CFNP
Teaching Specialist
School of Nursing
University of Minnesota
Twin Cities, Minnesota

Cynthia Blank-Reid, RN, MSN, CEN
Trauma Clinical Nurse Specialist
Temple University Hospital
Philadelphia, Pennsylvania
Clinical Adjunct Associate Professor
Drexel University College of Nursing and
    Health Professions
Philadelphia, Pennsylvania

Elizabeth Blunt, PhD (c), MSN
Assistant Professor and Director,
    Graduate Nursing Programs
Drexel University College of Nursing and
    Health Professions
Philadelphia, Pennsylvania

Margaret Brenner, RN, MSN
Senior Consultant, Pinnacle Healthcare
    Group, Inc.
Paoli, Pennsylvania

Margaret Brogan, RN, BSN
Registered Nurse/Expert
Children's Memorial Hospital
Chicago, Illinois

Mary Lynn Burnett, RN, PhD
Assistant Professor of Nursing
Wichita State University
Wichita, Kansas

Corine K. Carlson, RN, MS
Assistant Professor
Department of Nursing
Luther College
Decorah, Iowa

Nancy Clarkson, MEd, RN, BC
Professor and Chairperson
Department of Nursing
Finger Lakes Community College
Canandaigua, New York

Nancy Clarkson, RN, C, MEd
Associate Professor of Nursing
Finger Lakes Community College
Canandaigua, New York

Gretchen Reising Cornell, RN, PhD, CNE
Professor of Nursing
Utah Valley State College
Orem, Utah

Vera V. Cull, RN, DSN
Former Assistant Professor of Nursing
University of Alabama
Birmingham, Alabama

Deborah L. Dalrymple, RN, MSN, CRNI
Associate Professor of Nursing
Montgomery County Community College
Blue Bell, Pennsylvania

Laura DeHelian, RN, PhD, APRN, BC
Former Assistant Professor of Nursing
Cleveland State University
Cleveland, Ohio

ix

Della J. Derscheid, RN, MS, CNS
Assistant Professor
Department of Nursing
Mayo Clinic
Mayo Clinic College of Nursing
Rochester, Minnesota

Judy Donlen, RN, DNSc
Executive Director, Southern New Jersey
Perinatal Cooperative
Pennsauken, New Jersey

Judith L. Draper, APRN, BC
Assistant Professor
Drexel University College of Nursing and
   Health Professions
Philadelphia, Pennsylvania

Theresa M. Fay-Hillier, MSN, RN, CS
Adjunct Faculty
Drexel University College of Nursing and
   Health Professions
Philadelphia, Pennsylvania

Marcia R. Gardner, MA, RN, CPNP, CPN
Assistant Professor
Drexel University College of Nursing and
   Health Professions
Philadelphia, Pennsylvania

Ann Garey, MSN, APRN, BC, FNP
Carle Foundation Hospital
Urbana, Illinois

Jeanne Gelman, RN, MA, MSN
Professor Emeritus, Psychiatric-Mental
   Health Nursing
Widener University
Chester, Pennsylvania

Theresa M. Giglio, RD, MS
Instructor, LaSalle University
Philadelphia, Pennsylvania

Beth Good, RN, MSN, BSN
Teaching Specialist
University of Minnesota
Minneapolis, Minnesota

Samantha Grover, RN, BSN, CNS
Psychiatric Mental Health Clinical
   Specialist
MeritCare Health System
Moorhead, Minnesota

Judith M. Hall, RNC, MSN, IBCLC, LCCE
Lactation Consultant and Childbirth
   Educator
Mary Washington Hospital
Fredericksburg, Virginia

**Judith M. Hall, RNC, MSN, IBCLC,
LCCE, FACCE**
Mary Washington Hospital
Fredericksburg, Virginia

**Jeanne M. Harkness, RN, BA, MSN,
BSN, AOCN**
Clinical Practice Specialist
Jane Brattain Breast Center
Park Nicollet Clinic
St. Louis Park, Minnesota

Marilyn Herbert-Ashton, RN, C, MS
Director, Wellness Center
F. F. Thompson Health Systems, Inc.
Adjunct Professor of Nursing
Finger Lakes Community College
Canandaigua, New York

Marilyn Herbert-Ashton, MS, RN, BC
Virginia Western Community College
Roanoke, VA

Holly Hillman, RN, MSN
Assistant Professor
Montgomery County Community College
Blue Bell, Pennsylvania

Lorraine C. Igo, RN, MSN, EdD
Assistant Professor
Drexel University College of Nursing and
   Health Professions
Philadelphia, Pennsylvania

Linda Irle, RN, MSN, APN, CNP
Coordinator, Maternal-Child Nursing
University of Illinois
Urbana, Illinois
Family Nurse Practitioner, Acute Care,
Carle Clinic,
Champaign, Illinois

Amy Jacobson, RN, BA
Staff Nurse
United Hospital
St. Paul, Minnesota

Nancy H. Jacobson, MSN, APRN-BC, CS
Staff Development Coordinator
Rydal Park
Rydal, Pennsylvania

Nancy H. Jacobson, RN, CS, MSN
Senior Manager
The Whitman Group
Huntington Valley, Pennsylvania

Nadine James, RN, PhD
Assistant Professor of Nursing
University of Southern Mississippi
Hattiesburg, Mississippi

Lisa Jensen, CS, MS, APRN
Salt Lake City VA Healthcare System
Salt Lake City, Utah

Ellen Joswiak, RN, MA
Assistant Professor of Nursing
Staff Nurse
Mayo Medical Center
Rochester, Minnesota

Charlotte D. Kain, RN, C, EdD
Professor Nursing, Health Care of Women
Montgomery County Community College
Blue Bell, Pennsylvania

Roseann Tirotta Kaplan, MSN, RN, CS
Adjunct Faculty
Drexel University College of Nursing and
   Health Professions
Philadelphia, Pennsylvania

Betsy Ann Skrha Kennedy, RN, MS, CS, LCCE
Nursing Instructor
Rochester Community and Technical
   College
Rochester, Minnesota

Robin M. Lally, PhD, RN, BA, AOCN, CNS
Teaching Specialist; Office 6-155
School of Nursing
University of Minnesota
Twin Cities, Minnesota

Penny Leake, RN, PhD
Luther College
Decorah, Iowa

Barbara Mandleco, RN, PhD
Associate Professor & Undergraduate
   Program Coordinator
College of Nursing
Brigham Young University
Provo, Utah

Mary Lou Manning, RN, PhD, CPNP
Director, Infection Control and
   Occupational Health
The Children's Hospital of Philadelphia
Adjunct Assistant Professor
University of Pennsylvania School of
   Nursing
Philadelphia, Pennsylvania

Gerry Matsumura, RN, PhD, MSN, BSN
Former Associate Professor of Nursing
Brigham Young University
Provo, Utah

Alberta McCaleb, RN, DSN
Associate Professor
Chair, Undergraduate Studies
University of Alabama School of Nursing
University of Alabama at Birmingham
Birmingham, Alabama

Judith C. Miller, RN, MSN
President, Nursing Tutorial and
   Consulting Services
Clifton, Virginia

Eileen Moran, RN, C, MSN
Clinical Educator
Abington Memorial Hospital
Abington, Pennsylvania

JoAnn Mulready-Shick, RN, MS
Dean, Nursing and Allied Health
Roxbury Community College
Boston, Massachusetts

Patricia Murdoch, RN, MS
Nurse Practitioner
University of Illinois, Chicago
Urbana, Illinois

Jayme S. Nelson, RN, MS, ARNP-C
Adult Nurse Practitioner
Assistant Professor of Nursing
Luther College
Decorah, Iowa

Janice Nuuhiwa, MSN, CPON, APN/CNS
Staff Development Specialist
Hematology/Oncology/Stem Cell
Transplant Division
Children's Memorial Hospital
Chicago, Illinois

Kristen L. Osborn, MSN, CRNP
Pediatric Nurse Specialist
UAB School of Nursing
UAB Pediatric Hematology/Oncology
Birmingham, Alabama

Marie O'Toole, RN, EdD
Associate Professor, College of Nursing
Rutgers, The State University of New Jersey
Newark, New Jersey

Faye A. Pearlman, RN, MSN, MBA
Assistant Professor
Drexel University College of Nursing and
Health Professions
Philadelphia, Pennsylvania

Karen D. Peterson, RN, MSN, BSN, PNP
Pediatric Nurse Practitioner
Division of Endocrinology
Children's Memorial Hospital
Chicago, Illinois

Kristin Sandau, RN, PhD
Bethel University's Department of
Nursing
United's John Nasseff Heart Hospital
Minneapolis, Minnesota

Elizabeth Sawyer, RN, BSN, CCRN
Registered Nurse
United Hospital
St. Paul, Minnesota

Lisa A. Seldomridge, RN, PhD
Associate Professor of Nursing
Salisbury University
Salisbury, Maryland

Janice Selekman, RN, DNSc
Professor and Chair
Department of Nursing
University of Delaware
Newark, Delaware

Robert Shearer, CRNA, MSN
Assistant Professor
Drexel University College of Nursing and
Health Professions
Philadelphia, Pennsylvania

Constance O. Kolva Taylor, RN, MSN
Kolva Consulting
Harrisburg, Pennsylvania

Magdeleine Vasso, MSN, RN
Assistant Professor
Drexel University College of Nursing and
Health Professions
Philadelphia, Pennsylvania

Janice L. Vincent, RN, DSN
University of Alabama School of Nursing
University of Alabama at Birmingham
Birmingham, Alabama

Margaret Vogel, RN, MSN, BSN
Nursing Instructor
Rochester Community & Technical
College
Rochester, Minnesota

Anne Robin Waldman, RN, C, MSN, AOCN
Clinical Nurse Specialist
Albert Einstein Medical Center
Philadelphia, Pennsylvania

Mary Shannon Ward, RN, MSN
Children's Memorial Hospital
Chicago, Illinois

Virginia R. Wilson, RN, MSN, CEN
Assistant Professor, Graduate Nursing
Programs
Drexel University College of Nursing and
Health Professions
Philadelphia, Pennsylvania

Preface

Congratulations on discovering the best new review series for the NCLEX-RN®! Thomson Delmar Learning's Nursing Review Series is designed to maximize your study in the core subject areas covered on the NCLEX-RN® examination. The series consists of 8 books:

Pharmacology

Medical-Surgical Nursing

Pediatric Nursing

Maternity and Women's Health Nursing

Gerontologic Nursing

Psychiatric Nursing

Legal and Ethical Nursing

Community Health Nursing

Each text has been developed expressly to meet your needs as you study and prepare for the all-important licensure examination. Taking this exam is a stressful event and constitutes a major career milestone. Passing the NCLEX is the key to your future ability to practice as a registered nurse.

Each text in the series is designed around the most current test plan for the NCLEX-RN® and provides a focused and complete content review in each subject area. Additionally, there are up to 400 review questions in each text: questions at the end of most every chapter and three 100 question review tests that support the chapter content. Each set of review questions is followed by answers and rationales for both the right and wrong answers. There is also a free PDA download of review questions available with the purchase of any of these review texts! It is this combination of content review and self assessment that provides a powerful learning experience for you as you prepare for you examination.

ORGANIZATION

Thomson Delmar Learning's unique Pharmacology review book provides you with an intensive review in this all important subject area. Drugs are grouped by classification and similarities to aid you in consolidating this pertinent but sometimes overwhelming information. Included in this text are:

- A section on herbal medicines, now being tested on the exam.
- Case studies that apply relevant drug content
- Prototypes for most drug classifications
- Mechanism of drug action
- Uses and adverse effects
- Nursing implications and discharge teaching
- Related drugs and their variance from the prototype

The review texts for Medical-Surgical Nursing, Pediatric Nursing, Maternity Nursing, Gerontological Nursing and Psychiatric Nursing follow a systematic approach that includes:

- The nursing process integrated with a body systems approach
- Introductory review of normal anatomy and physiology as well as basic theories and principles
- Review of pertinent disorders for each system including: general characteristics, pathophysiology/psychopathology
- Medical management
- Assessment data
- Nursing interventions and client education

Community Health Nursing and Legal and Ethical Nursing are unique review texts in the marketplace. They include aspects of community health nursing and legal/ethical subject matter that is covered on the NCLEX-RN® exam. Community Health topics covered are: case management, long-term care, home health care and hospice. Legal and ethical topics include: cultural diversity, leadership and management, ethical issues and legal issues for older adults.

FEATURES

All questions in each text in the series are compliant with the most current test plan from the National Council of State Boards of Nursing (NCSBN). All questions are followed by answers and rationales for both right and wrong choices. Included are many of the alternative format questions first introduced to the exam in 2003. An icon identifies these alternate types ⊙. The questions in each of these texts are written primarily at the application or analysis cognitive levels allowing you to further enhance critical thinking skills which are heavily weighted on the NCLEX.

In addition, with the purchase of any of these texts, a free PDA download is available to you. It provides you with up to an additional 225 questions with which you can practice your test taking skills.

Thomson Delmar Learning is committed to help you reach your fullest professional potential. Good luck on the NCLEX-RN® examination!

> To access your free PDA download for Thomson Delmar Learning's Nursing Review Series visit the online companion resource at **www.delmarhealthcare.com** Click on Online Companions then select the Nursing discipline.

Reviewers

Judy Bourrand, RN, MSN
Ida V. Moffett School of Nursing
Samford University
Birmingham, Alabama

Mary Kathie Doyle, BS, CCRN,
Instructor
Maria College
Troy, New York

Mary Lashley, PhD, RN, CS
Associate Professor
Towson University
Towson, Maryland

Melissa Lickteig, EdD, RN
Instructor, School of Nursing
Georgia Southern University
Statesboro, Georgia

Darlene Mathis, MSN, RN APRN, BC,
NP-C, CRNP
Assistant Professor
Ida V. Moffett School of Nursing
Samford University
Birmingham, Alabama

Barbara McGraw, MSN, RN
Instructor
Central Community College
Grand Island, Nebraska

Carol Meadows, MNSc, RNP, APN
Eleanor Mann School of Nursing
University of Arkansas
Fayetteville, Arkansas

Maria Smith, DSN, RN, CCRN
Professor, School of Nursing
Middle Tennessee State University
Murfreesboro, Tennessee

Introduction

Charlotte D. Kain, RNC, EdD
Judith M. Hall, RNC, MSN, IBCLC, LCCE, FACCE

This section covers the health care needs of females from adolescence through late adulthood. Emphasis is placed on the childbearing cycle and the normal neonate, and frequently encountered health care problems. Cultural differences are addressed.

The unit begins with a review of the anatomy and physiology of the female reproductive system as a basis for understanding the entire childbearing process. Nursing process is emphasized throughout, and nursing diagnoses are used to identify the client's health care needs and to select nursing interventions.

Nursing process always must be implemented with an awareness of the interrelationship, during childbearing, of the maternal and fetal needs and their manifestations. The nurse needs to keep in mind that interventions for the mother may have an impact on the developing fetus, and vice versa. Medications for maternal conditions may affect the fetus, and fetal distress may require that the mother undergo surgery.

In this unit, a major assertion is that childbearing, for most women, is a normal, healthy life event. Discomforts and complications of childbearing also are covered, and these conditions are presented after the content that reviews the natural progression of events in pregnancy and childbearing. In this manner, the factors that alter pregnancy from a normal life event to a life crisis can be clearly identified.

In addition to childbearing, the unit includes a review of frequently encountered health care conditions of women. These conditions usually involve the reproductive system or its accessory organs and include normally occurring states, such as menopause, as well as pathologic conditions, such as gynecologic cancer.

1

Overview of Anatomy and Physiology of the Female Reproductive System

■ ANATOMY

External Structures

See Figure 1-1.

A. *Mons veneris*: rounded, soft, fatty, and loose connective tissue over the symphysis pubis. Dark, curly pubic hair growth in typical triangular shape begins here 1 to 2 years before the onset of menstruation.

B. *Labia majora*: lengthwise fatty folds of skin extending from the mons to the perineum that protect the labia minora, the urinary meatus, and the vaginal introitus.

C. *Labia minora*: thinner, lengthwise folds of hairless skin, extending from the clitoris to the fourchette.
   1. Glands in the labia minora lubricate the vulva.
   2. The labia minora are very sensitive because of their rich nerve supply.
   3. The space between the labia minora is called the vestibule.

D. *Clitoris*: small erectile organ located beneath the arch of the pubis, containing more nerve endings than the glans penis; sensitive to temperature and touch; secretes a fatty substance called smegma.

E. *Vestibule*: area formed by the labia minora, clitoris, and fourchette, enclosing the openings to the urethra and vagina, Skene's and Bartholin's glands; easily irritated by chemicals, discharges, or friction.
   1. *Urethra*: external opening to the urinary bladder
   2. *Skene's glands* (also called *paraurethral glands*): secrete a small amount of mucus; especially susceptible to infections
   3. *Bartholin's glands*: located on either side of the vaginal orifice; secrete clear mucus during sexual arousal; susceptible to infection, as well as cyst and abscess formation
   4. *Vaginal orifice* and *hymen*: elastic, partial fold of tissue surrounding opening to the vagina

F. *Fourchette*: thin fold of tissue formed by the merging of the labia majora and labia minora, below the vaginal orifice.

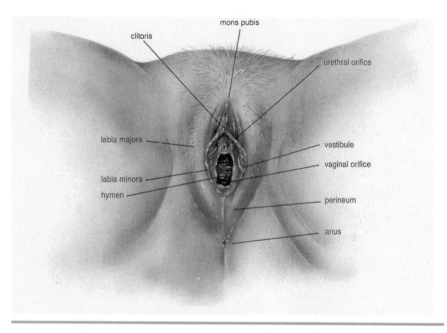

FIGURE 1-1   External structures of the female reproductive system

G. *Perineum*: muscular, skin-covered area between vaginal opening and anus.
  1.   Underlying the perineum are the paired muscle groups that form the supportive "sling" for the pelvic organs, capable of great distension during the birth process.
  2.   An episiotomy can be made in the perineum if necessary during the birth process.

Internal Structures

See Figure 1-2.
A. *Fallopian tubes*: paired tubules extending from the cornu of the uterus to the ovaries that serve as the passageway for the ova. Mucosal lining of tubes resembles that of vagina and uterus; therefore, infection may extend from lower organs.
B. *Uterus*: hollow, pear-shaped muscular organ, freely movable in pelvic cavity, comprised of *fundus, corpus, isthmus*, and *cervix*. Cervix has internal and external os, separated by the cervical canal. Wall of uterus has three layers.
  1.   *Endometrium*: inner layer, highly vascular, shed during menstruation and following delivery
  2.   *Myometrium*: middle layer, comprised of smooth muscle fibers running in three directions; expels fetus during birth process, then contracts around blood vessels to prevent hemorrhage
  3.   *Parietal peritoneum*: serous outer layer

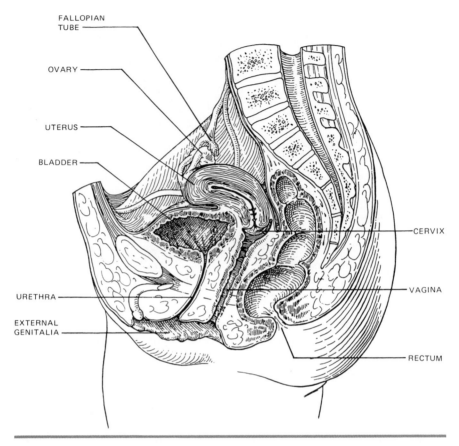

FALLOPIAN TUBE
OVARY
UTERUS
BLADDER
CERVIX
VAGINA
URETHRA
EXTERNAL GENITALIA
RECTUM

FIGURE 1-2   Internal structures of the female reproductive system

C. *Ovaries*: oval, almond-sized organs on either side of the uterus that produce ova and hormones.
D. *Vagina*: Muscular, distensible tube connecting perineum and cervix; the birth canal.

The Pelvis

Right and left innominate bones, sacrum, and coccyx form the bony passage through which the baby passes during birth. Relationship between pelvic size/ shape and baby may affect labor or make vaginal delivery impossible.
A. Pelvic measurements
    1. True conjugate: from upper margin of symphysis pubis to sacral promontory, should be at least 11 cm; may be obtained by X-ray or ultrasound.

2. Diagonal conjugate: from lower border of symphysis pubis to sacral promontory; should be 12.5-13 cm; may be obtained by vaginal examination.
3. Obstetric conjugate: from inner surface of symphysis pubis, slightly below upper border, to sacral promontory, it is the *most important pelvic measurement*; can be estimated by subtracting 1.5-2 cm from diagonal conjugate.
4. Intertuberous diameter: measures the outlet between the inner borders of the ischial tuberosities; should be at least 8 cm.

B. Pelvic shapes
1. Android: narrow, heart shaped; male-type pelvis
2. Anthropoid: narrow, oval shaped; resembles ape pelvis
3. Gynecoid: classic female pelvis; wide and well rounded in all directions
4. Platypelloid: wide but flat; may still allow vaginal delivery

C. Pelvic divisions
1. False pelvis: shallow upper basin of the pelvis; supports the enlarging uterus, but not important obstetrically
2. Linea terminalis: plane dividing upper or false pelvis from lower or true pelvis
3. True pelvis: consists of the pelvic inlet, pelvic cavity, and pelvic outlet. Measurements of true pelvis influence the conduct and progress of labor and delivery.

The Breasts

A. Paired mammary glands on the anterior chest wall, between the second and sixth ribs, comprised of glandular tissue, fat, and connective tissue.
B. Nipple and areola are darker in color than breasts.
C. Responsible for lactation after delivery.

■ PHYSIOLOGY

Menarche

Onset of the menstrual cycle; puberty.

Menstrual Cycle

See Figure 1-3.
A. Complex pituitary/ovarian/uterine interaction.
B. Controls ripening and release of an ovum on a regular basis, and preparation for its fertilization and implantation in a thickened uterine lining (endometrium).
C. When fertilization/implantation do not occur, the endometrium is shed (menstruation), and the cycle begins again, due to follicle-stimulating hormone (FSH) and luteinizing hormone (LH) from the anterior pituitary.

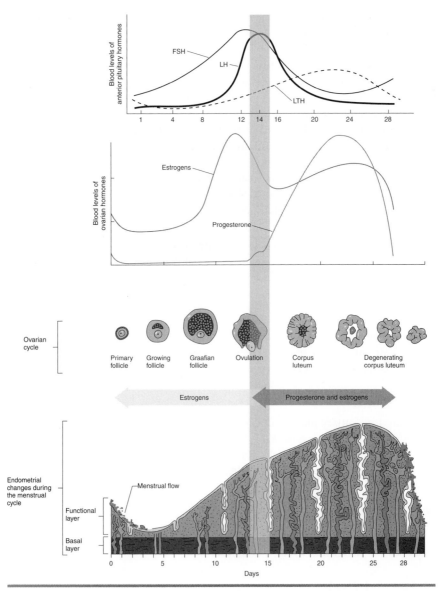

FIGURE 1-3   Menstrual cycle illustrating the levels of pituitary and ovarian hormones, ovarian cycle, and endometrial changes

D. Stages of cycle
   1. *Menstruation*: first days of cycle when endometrium is shed.
   2. *Proliferative phase*: major hormone involved is estrogen, which influences build-up of endometrium; also called *follicular phase*.

3. *Ovulation*: release of ovum, usually 14 days (plus or minus 2) before end of cycle.
4. *Secretory phase*: major hormone is progesterone, which influences myometrium (decreased irritability); also called *luteal phase*.

Menopause (Climacteric)

A. Decline in ovarian function and hormone production.
B. Characterized by menstrual cycle irregularity and, in some women, by vasomotor instability and loss of bone density.

Sexual Response in the Female: Four Phases

A. Excitement phase: vaginal lubrication and vasocongestion of external genitals.
B. Plateau phase: formation of orgasmic platform in vagina.
C. Orgasmic phase: strong rhythmic contractions of vagina and uterus.
D. Resolution phase: cervix dips into seminal pool in vagina; all organs return to previous condition.

2

The Childbearing Cycle

■ CONCEPTION

See Figure 2-1.

A. The penetration of one ovum (female gamete) by one sperm (male gamete), resulting in a fertilized ovum (zygote). Each gamete has haploid number of chromosomes (23). Zygote has diploid number (46) with one of each pair from each parent.

B. Sex of child is determined at moment of conception by male gamete. If X-bearing male gamete unites with ovum, result is a female child (X + X). If Y-bearing male gamete unites with ovum, result is a male child (X + Y).

C. Usually occurs in the outer third of the fallopian tube.

D. Multiple pregnancies result from
   1. Two or more fertilized ova (fraternal or dizygotic)
   2. Single fertilized ovum that divides—always same sex, only 1 chorion (identical or monozygotic)

■ NIDATION (IMPLANTATION)

A. Burrowing of developing zygote into endometrial lining of uterus.

B. May take place 7–10 days after fertilization, while zygote develops to trophoblastic stage.

C. Chorionic villi appear on surface of trophoblast and secrete human chorionic gonadotropin (HCG), which inhibits ovulation during pregnancy by stimulating continuous production of estrogen and progesterone. This secretion of HCG forms the basis of the various tests for pregnancy.

■ DEVELOPMENTAL STAGES

Fertilized Ovum

A. From conception through first 2 weeks of pregnancy.

B. Nidation complete by the end of this period.

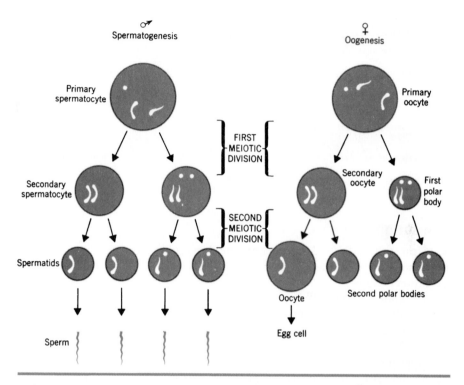

FIGURE 2-1   Spermatogenesis and oogenesis. A primary spermatocyte produces four sperm, but only one egg results from meiosis of a primary oocyte. The polar bodies are functionless.

Embryo

A. From end of second week through end of eighth week (also called period of organogenesis).

B. Critical time in development; embryo most vulnerable to teratogens (harmful substances or conditions), which can result in congenital anomalies.

Fetus

A. From end of eighth week to termination of pregnancy.

B. Continued maturation of already-formed organ systems.

■ SPECIAL STRUCTURES OF PREGNANCY

Fetal Membranes

A. Arise from the zygote.

B. Inner (amnion) and outer (chorion).

C. Hold the developing fetus as well as the amniotic fluid.

NURSING ALERT

An ovum is receptive to fertilization for only 24–48 hours after ovulation.

NURSING ALERT

The zygote's sex is determined at the moment of fertilization.

Amniotic Fluid

A. Clear, yellowish fluid surrounding the developing fetus.
B. Average amount 1000 ml.
C. Protects fetus.
   1. Allows free movement.
   2. Maintains temperature.
   3. Provides oral fluid.
D. Can be aspirated and tested for various diseases and abnormalities during pregnancy.
E. Alkaline pH: can be tested when membranes rupture to distinguish from urine.

Umbilical Cord

A. Connecting link between fetus and placenta.
B. Contains two arteries and one vein supported by mucoid material (Wharton's jelly) to prevent kinking and knotting.
C. There are no pain receptors in the umbilical cord.

Placenta

See Figure 2-2.
A. Transient organ allowing passage of nutrients and waste materials between mother and fetus.
B. Also acts as an endocrine organ and as a sieve which allows smaller particles through and holds back larger molecules. Passage of materials in either direction is effected by:
   1. Diffusion: gases, water, electrolytes.
   2. Facilitated transfer: glucose, amino acids, minerals.
   3. Pinocytosis: movement of minute particles (e.g., fats).
   4. Leakage: caused by membrane defect; may allow maternal and fetal blood mixing.

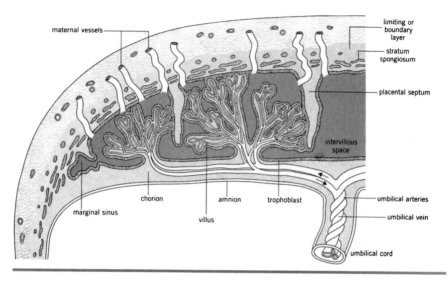

FIGURE 2-2 Placental circulation. Through the placenta the fetus gets nourishment and excretes waste.

C. Mother also transmits immunoglobulin G (IgG) to fetus through placenta, providing limited passive immunity.
D. Hormones produced by the placenta include
   1. HCG: early in pregnancy, responsible for continued action of corpus luteum, is basis of pregnancy tests.
   2. Human chorionic somato-mammotropin/human placental lactogen (HCS/HPL): similar to growth hormone; affects maternal insulin production; prepares breasts for lactation.
   3. Estrogen and progesterone: necessary for continuation of pregnancy.

Fetal Circulation

A. Arteries in cord and fetal body carry deoxygenated blood.
B. Vein in cord and those in fetal body carry oxygenated blood.
C. Ductus venosus connects umbilical vein and inferior vena cava; bypassing portal circulation; closes after birth.
D. Foramen ovale allows blood to flow from right atrium to left atrium, bypassing lungs. Closes functionally at birth because of increased pressure in left atrium; anatomic closure may take several weeks to several months.
E. Ductus arteriosus allows blood flow from pulmonary artery to aorta, bypassing fetal lungs; closes after delivery.

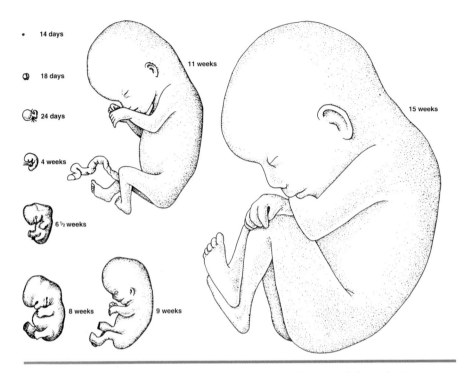

FIGURE 2-3 Changes in the body size of the embryo and fetus during development in the uterus (all figures are natural size)

Fetal Growth and Development

A. Organ systems develop from three primary germ layers.
   1. Ectoderm: outer layer, produces skin, nails, nervous system, and tooth enamel.
   2. Mesoderm: middle layer, produces connective tissue, muscles, blood, and circulatory system.
   3. Endoderm: inner layer, produces linings of gastrointestinal and respiratory tracts, endocrine glands, and auditory canal.
B. Timetable (Figure 2-3 and Table 2-1).
C. Measurements of length of pregnancy
   1. Days: 267–280
   2. Weeks: 40, plus or minus 2
   3. Months (lunar): 10
   4. Months (calendar): 9
   5. Trimesters: 3
D. Estimated due date/estimated date of confinement (*Nägele's rule*); see Figure 2-4. This calculation is an estimation only. Most women deliver: due date + or − 2 weeks. Sonogram dating used to confirm dates.

TABLE 2-1 Markers in Fetal Development

Date*	Development
4 weeks	All systems in rudimentary form; heart chambers formed and heart is beating. Embryo length about 0.4 cm; weight about 0.4 g.
8 weeks	Some distinct features in face; head large in proportion to rest of body; some movement. Length about 2.5 cm, weight 2 g.
12 weeks	Sex distinguishable; ossification in most bones; kidneys secrete urine; able to suck and swallow. Length 6–8 cm, weight 19 g.
16 weeks	More human appearance; earliest movement likely to be felt by mother; meconium in bowel; scalp hair develops. Length 11.5–13.5 cm, weight 100 g.
20 weeks	Vernix caseosa and lanugo appear; movement usually felt by mother; heart rate audible; bones hardening. Length 16–18.5 cm, weight 300 g.
24 weeks	Body well proportioned; skin red and wrinkled; hearing established. Length 23 cm, weight 600 g.
28 weeks	Infant viable, but immature if born at this time. Body less wrinkled; appearance of nails. Length 27 cm, weight 1100 g.
32 weeks	Subcutaneous fat beginning to deposit; L/S ratio in lungs now 1.2:1; skin smooth and pink. Length 31 cm, weight 1800–2100 g.
36 weeks	Lanugo disappearing; body usually plump; L/S ratio usually 2:1; definite sleep/wake cycle. Length 35 cm, weight 2200–2900 g.
40 weeks	Full-term pregnancy. Baby is active, with good muscle tone; strong suck reflex; if male, testes in scrotum; little lanugo. Length 40 cm, weight 3200 g or more.

*Dates are approximate, but developmental level should have been reached by the end of the time period specified.

- Add 7 days to the first day of the last normal menstrual period
- Subtract 3 months
- Add 1 year

Example: 1st day of LNMP = September 16, 1998
                        Add 7 days = September 23
                Subtract 3 months = June 23
                        Add 1 year = June 23, 1999, will be
                                        estimated due date

FIGURE 2-4   Nägele's rule

■ PHYSICAL AND PSYCHOLOGIC CHANGES OF PREGNANCY

Reproductive System

A. External structures: enlarged due to increased vascularity.

B. Ovaries
1. No ovulation during pregnancy
2. Corpus luteum persists in early pregnancy until development of placenta is complete

C. Fallopian tubes: elongate as uterus rises in pelvic and abdominal cavities.

D. Vagina
1. Increased vascularity (*Chadwick's sign*)
2. Estrogen-induced leukorrhea
3. Change in pH (less acidic) may favor overgrowth of yeastlike organisms
4. Connective tissue loosens in preparation for distention of labor and delivery.

E. Cervix
1. Softens and loosens in preparation for labor and delivery (*Goodell's sign*).
2. Mucous production increases, and plug (operculum) is formed as bacterial barricade.

F. Uterus
1. Hypertrophy and hyperplasia of muscle cells
2. Development of fibroelastic tissue that increases ability to contract
3. Shape changes from pearlike to ovoid
4. Rises out of pelvic cavity by 16th week of pregnancy
5. Increased vascularity and softening of isthmus (*Hegar's sign*)
6. Mild contractions (*Braxton Hicks' sign*) beginning in the fourth month through end of pregnancy

G. Breasts
1. Increased vascularity, sensitivity, and fullness
2. Nipples and areola darken
3. Nipples become more erectile
4. Proliferation of ducts and alveolar tissue evidenced by increased breast size
5. Production of colostrum by the second trimester

Cardiovascular System

A. Blood volume expands as much as 50% to meet demands of new tissue and increased needs of all systems.

B. Progesterone relaxes smooth muscle, resulting in vasodilation and accommodation of increased volume.

C. RBC volume increases as much as 30%; may be slight decline in hematocrit as pregnancy progresses because of this relative imbalance (physiologic anemia).

D. Stroke volume and cardiac output increase.

E. WBCs increase.

F. Greater tendency to coagulation.

G. Blood pressure may drop in early pregnancy; should not rise during last half of pregnancy.

H. Heart rate increases; palpitations possible.

I. Blood flow to uterus and placenta is maximized by side-lying position.

J. Varicosities may occur in vulva and rectum as well as lower extremities.

Respiratory System

A. Increased vascularity of mucous membranes of this system gives rise to symptoms of nasal and pharyngeal congestion and fullness in the ears.

B. Shape of thorax shortens and widens to accommodate the growing fetus.

C. Slight increase in respiratory rate.

D. Dyspnea may occur at end of third trimester before engagement or "lightening."

E. Increased respiratory volume by 40 to 50%.

F. Oxygen consumption increases by 15%.

Renal System

A. Kidney filtration rate increases as much as 50%.

B. Glucose threshold drops; sodium threshold rises.

C. Water retention increases as pregnancy progresses.

D. Enlarging uterus causes pressure on bladder resulting in frequency of urination, especially during first trimester; later in pregnancy relaxed ureters are displaced laterally, increasing possibility of stasis and infection.

E. Presence of protein (not an expected component of maternal urine) indicates possible renal disease or pregnancy-induced hypertension.

Integumentary System

A. Increased pigmentation of nipples and areolas.

B. Possible appearance of *chloasma* (mask of pregnancy): darkening of areas on forehead and cheekbones.

C. Appearance of *linea nigra*, darkened line bisecting abdomen from symphysis pubis to top of fundus.
D. Striae (stretch marks): separation of underlying connective tissue in breasts, abdomen, thighs, and buttocks; fade after delivery.
E. Greater sweat and sebaceous gland activity.

Musculoskeletal System

A. Alterations in posture and walking gait caused by change in center of gravity as pregnancy progresses.
B. Increased joint mobility as a result of action of ovarian hormone (relaxin) on connective tissue.
C. Possible backache.
D. Occasional cramps in calf may occur with hypocalcemia.

Neurologic System

A. Few changes with a typical pregnancy.
B. Pressure on sciatic nerve may occur later in pregnancy due to fetal position.

Gastrointestinal System

A. Bleeding gums and hypersalivation may occur.
B. Tooth loss due to demineralization should *not* occur.
C. Nausea and vomiting in first trimester due to rising levels of HCG.
D. Appetite usually improves.
E. Cravings or desires for strange food combinations may occur.
F. Progesterone-induced relaxation of muscle tone leads to slow movement of food through GI tract; may result in heartburn.
G. Constipation may occur as water is reabsorbed in large intestine.
H. Emptying time for gallbladder may be prolonged; increased incidence of gallstones.

Endocrine System

A. Pituitary: FSH and LH greatly decreased; oxytocin secreted during labor and after delivery; prolactin responsible for initiation and continuation of lactation.
B. Progesterone secreted by corpus luteum until formation of placenta.
C. Principal source of estrogen is placenta, synthesized from fetal precursors.
D. HCS/HPL produced by placenta; similar to growth hormone, it prepares breasts for lactation; also affects insulin/glucose metabolism. May overstress maternal pancreas.
E. Ovaries secrete relaxin during pregnancy.
F. Slight increase in thyroid activity and basal metabolic rate (BMR).

G. Pancreas may be stressed due to complex interaction of glucose metabolism, HCS/HPL, and cortisol, resulting in diminished effectiveness of insulin, and demand for increased production.

Psychosocial Changes

A. First trimester
   1. Mother needs accurate diagnosis of pregnancy.
   2. Works through characteristic ambivalence of early pregnancy.
   3. Mother is self-centered, baby is "part" of her.
   4. Grandparents are usually the first relatives to be told of the pregnancy.
B. Second trimester
   1. Mother demonstrates growing realization of baby as separate and needing person.
   2. Fantasizes about unborn child.
C. Third trimester
   1. "Nesting" activity appears as due date approaches.
   2. Desire to be finished with pregnancy.
D. Anxiety over "safe passage" for self and baby through labor and delivery.
E. Reactions of father-to-be may parallel those of mother (e.g., ambivalence, anxiety). Additionally, as mother's pregnancy progresses he may experience similar physical changes.
F. Preparation of siblings varies according to their age and experience.

Transcultural Concerns in Pregnancy

A. Dominant philosophy concerning pregnancy and birth may differ in non-U.S. cultures. May view this as "healthy" time, with little or no insight concerning potential complications.
B. Biological variations may occur, e.g., higher rate of complications in women with sickle cell trait or gene; diabetes mellitus seen with more frequency in pregnant American Indians; increase in parasitic infections and hepatitis in women from Southeast Asia.
C. Behaviors during pregnancy (eating, sleeping, bathing, sexual activity, etc.) will differ from culture to culture.
D. Superstition, taboos, and "old wives' tales" may play an important role.
E. Most cultures consider childbirth to be the province of women; men's roles may be limited or excluded. This may include caregivers.
F. Perception of discomfort/pain will vary; may be influenced by cultural expectations as well as mother's own experiences.
G. Despite culture, many women prefer upright position for labor and birth, rather than lying down. Additionally, many women prefer to have the freedom to move around during labor, whenever possible.

H. After delivery, cultural rituals may refer to rest, seclusion, and purification. The postpartum women may be considered vulnerable. Applications of heat or cold, in air or water, need to be specially assessed.

I. Other areas of culturally related practices may be: nutrition, clothing, activity, resumption of contact with the community, resumption of sexual activities, and return to work.

J. Infant care (feeding, cord care, circumcision, clothing, sleeping arrangements) will vary among differing cultures.

K. Control of future fertility may vary from natural methods such as breastfeeding to the use of any available means.

The Antepartal Period

■ ASSESSMENT

Classification of Pregnancy

A. Gravida—number of times pregnant, regardless of duration, including the present pregnancy.
  1. Primagravida—pregnant for the first time
  2. Multigravida—pregnant for second or subsequent time

CHAPTER OUTLINE

Assessment

Analysis

Planning and Implementation

Evaluation

Complications of Pregnancy

Pre- and Coexisting Diseases of Pregnancy

B. Para—number of pregnancies that lasted more than 20 weeks, regardless of outcome.
  1. Nullipara—a woman who has not given birth to a baby beyond 20 weeks' gestation.
  2. Primipara—a woman who has given birth to one baby more than 20 weeks' gestation.
  3. Multipara—Woman who has had two or more births at more than 20 weeks' gestation · · · twins or triplets count as 1 para.
  4. TPAL—Para subdivided to reflect births that went to **T**erm, **P**remature births, **A**bortions, and **L**iving children.

Determination of Pregnancy

Diagnosis of pregnancy is based on pregnancy-related physical and hormonal changes and are classified as presumptive, probable, or positive.

Presumptive Signs and Symptoms (Subjective)

These changes may be noticed by the mother/health care provider but are *not* conclusive for pregnancy.
A. Amenorrhea (cessation of menstruation)
B. Nausea and vomiting
C. Urinary frequency
D. Fatigue
E. Breast changes
F. Weight change
G. Skin changes

H. Vaginal changes including leukorrhea
I. Quickening

Probable Signs and Symptoms (Objective)

These changes are usually noted by the health care provider but are *still not conclusive* for pregnancy.
A. Uterine enlargement
B. Changes in the uterus and cervix from increased vascularity
C. Ballottement: fetus rebounds against the examiner's hand when pushed gently upwards.
D. Braxton Hicks' contractions: occur early in pregnancy, although not usually sensed by the mother until the third trimester.
E. Laboratory tests for pregnancy
    1. Most tests rely on the presence of HCG in the blood or urine of the woman.
    2. Easy, inexpensive, but may give false readings with any handling error, medications, or detergent residue in laboratory equipment.
    3. Exception is the radioimmunoassay (RIA), which tests for the beta subunit of HCG and is considered to be so accurate as to be diagnostic for pregnancy.
F. Changes in skin pigmentation.

Positive Signs and Symptoms

These signs emanate from the fetus, are noted by the health care provider, and *are conclusive* for pregnancy.
A. Fetal heartbeat: detected as early as eighth week with an electronic device; after 16th week with a more conventional auscultory device.
B. Palpation of fetal outline.
C. Palpation of fetal movements.
D. Demonstration of fetal outline by either ultrasound (after sixth week) or X-ray (after 12th week).

■ ANALYSIS

Nursing diagnoses for the antepartal period *may* include
A. Deficient knowledge: information on the following topics needs to be given and reinforced
    1. Danger signals of pregnancy to be reported
    2. Dangerous behaviors during pregnancy (e.g., smoking, using drugs [especially alcohol], use of nonprescription medications)
B. In nutrition potential: individualized nutritional information will be needed
C. Activity intolerance: need for additional rest and benefits of a moderate exercise program
D. Anxiety
E. Risk for constipation

F. Disturbed body image
G. Ineffective coping
H. Powerlessness
I. Noncompliance
J. Risk for deficient fluid volume
K. Health-seeking behaviors

■ PLANNING AND IMPLEMENTATION
Goals

A. Establish a diagnosis of pregnancy.
B. Gather initial data to form the basis for comparison with data collected as pregnancy progresses.
C. Identify high-risk factors.
D. Propose realistic and necessary interventions.
E. Promote optimal health for mother and baby, providing any needed information.
F. Provide needed information for prepared childbirth.

Interventions

Prenatal Care

A. Time frame
  1. First visit: may be made as soon as woman suspects she is pregnant; frequently after first missed period.
  2. Subsequent visits: Every month until the 8th month, every 2 weeks during the 8th month, and weekly during the 9th month; more frequent visits are scheduled if problems arise.
B. Conduct of initial visit
  1. Extensive collection of data about client in all pertinent areas in order to form basis for comparison with data collected on subsequent visits and to screen for any high-risk factors
    a. Menstrual history: menarche, regularity, frequency and duration of flow, last period
    b. Obstetrical history: all pregnancies, complications, outcomes, contraceptive use, sexual history
    c. Medical history: include past illnesses, surgeries; current use of medications
    d. Family history/psychosocial data
    e. Information about the father-to-be may also be significant
    f. Current concerns
  2. Complete physical examination, including internal gynecologic exam and bimanual exam
  3. Laboratory work, including CBC, urinalysis, Pap test, blood type and Rh, rubella titer, testing for sexually transmitted diseases

(STD), other tests as indicated (e.g., TB test, hepatitis viral studies, EKG, etc.)

C. Conduct of subsequent visits
1. Continue collection of data, especially weight, blood pressure, urine screening for glucose and protein, evaluation of fetal development through auscultation of fetal heart rate (FHR) and palpation of fetal outline, measurement of fundal height as correlation for appropriate progress of pregnancy. Fundus palpable above symphysis at 12 weeks, at the level of umbilicus at 20 weeks, then approximately 1 cm per week until 36-38 weeks when head often descends and fundal measurement may drop somewhat.
2. Additional tests
   a. Hemoglobin and hematocrit 26–28 weeks
   b. Glucose screen 24–28 weeks
   c. Antibody screen at 28 weeks
   d. Beginning of 9th month, test for STDs, strep, other infections
3. Prepare for any necessary testing.
   a. Have client void (clean catch).
   b. Collect baseline data on vital signs.
   c. Collect specimen.
   d. Monitor client and fetus after procedure.
   e. Provide support to client.
   f. Document as needed.

Nutrition during Pregnancy

A. Weight gain
1. Variable, but 25 lb usually appropriate for average woman with single pregnancy.
2. Woman should have consistent, predictable pattern of weight gain, with only 2–3 lb in first trimester, then average 12 oz gain every week in second and third trimesters.
3. Gains mostly reflect maternal tissue in first half of pregnancy, and fetal tissue in second half of pregnancy.

B. Specific nutrient needs
1. *Calories*: usual addition is 300 kcal/day, but there will be specific guidelines for those beginning pregnancy either over- or underweight (never less than 1800 kcal/day).
2. *Protein*: additional 30 g/day to ensure intake of 74–76 g/day; very young pregnant adolescents and those with multiple pregnancies will need more protein.
3. *Carbohydrates*: intake must be sufficient for energy needs, using fresh fruits and vegetables as much as possible to derive additional fiber benefit; teach to avoid "empty" calories.

NURSING ALERT

Folic acid supplements are recommended during pregnancy to prevent neural tube defects.

NURSING ALERT

Lactating women should consume 3000 ml of fluids per day.

4. *Fats*: high-energy foods, which are needed to carry the fat-soluble vitamins.
5. *Iron*: needed by mother as well as fetus; reserves usually sufficient for first trimester, supplementation recommended after this time; iron preparations should be taken with source of vitamin C to promote absorption.
6. *Calcium*: 1200 mg per day needed; dairy products most frequent source, with supplementation for those with lactose intolerance.
7. *Sodium*: contained in most foods; needed in pregnancy; should not be restricted without serious indication.
8. *Vitamins*: both fat- and water-soluble are needed in pregnancy; essential for tissue growth and development, as well as regulation of metabolism. Generally not synthesized by body, nor stored in large amounts (folic acid special concern as deficiency may cause fetal anomalies and bleeding complications).
C. Dietary supplements: many health care providers supplement the pregnant woman's diet with an iron-fortified multivitamin to ensure essential levels.
D. Special concerns
   1. Religious, ethnic, and cultural practices that influence selection and preparation of foods
   2. Pica (ingestion of nonedible or nonnutritive substances)
   3. Vegan vegetarians—no meat products, may need B_{12} supplement
   4. Adolescence
   5. Economic deprivation
   6. Heavy smoking, alcohol consumption, drugs
   7. Previous reproductive problems

Education for Parenthood

A. Provision of information about pregnancy, labor and delivery, the postpartum period, and lactation.
B. Usually taught in small groups, may be individualized.

TABLE 3-1 Methods of Childbirth

Read method	The so-called natural childbirth method. Underlying concept: knowledge diminishes the fear that is key to pain. Classes include information as well as practice in relaxation and abdominal breathing techniques for labor.
Lamaze method	Psychoprophylactic method based on utilization of Pavlovian conditioned response theory. Classes teach replacement of usual response to pain with new, learned responses (breathing, effleurage, relaxation) in order to block recognition of pain and promote positive sense of control in labor.
Bradley method	Husband-coached childbirth. A modification of the Read method emphasizing working in harmony with the body.
Other methods	Hypnosis, yoga.

C. Topics can be grouped into early and late pregnancy, labor and delivery, and postdelivery/newborn care.
D. Emphasis placed on both physical and psychosocial changes seen in childbearing cycle.
E. Preparation for childbirth: intended to provide knowledge and alternative coping behaviors in order to diminish anxiety and discomfort, and promote cooperation with the birth process; see Table 3-1 for specific methodologies.

Determination of Fetal Status and Risk Factors
A. Fetal diagnostic tests
　1. Used to
　　a. Identify or confirm the existence of risk factor(s)
　　b. Validate pregnancy
　　c. Observe progress of pregnancy
　　d. Identify optimum time for induction of labor if indicated
　　e. Identify genetic abnormalities
　2. Types
　　a. *Chorionic villi sampling (CVS)*: earliest test possible on fetal cells (9-12 weeks); sample obtained by slender catheter passed through cervix to implantation site.
　　b. *Ultrasound*: use of sound and returning echo patterns to identify intrabody structures. Useful early in pregnancy to identify

gestational sac(s) and to assist in pregnancy dating. Later uses include assessment of fetal viability, growth patterns, anomalies, fluid volume, uterine anomalies, and adnexal masses. Used as an adjunct to amniocentesis; safe for fetus (no ionizing radiation).

   c. *Amniocentesis*: location and aspiration of amniotic fluid for examination; possible after the 14th week when sufficient amounts are present. Used to identify chromosomal aberrations, sex of fetus, levels of alphafetoprotein and other chemicals indicative of neural tube defects and inborn errors of metabolism, gestational age, Rh factor.

   d. *X-ray*: can be used late in pregnancy (after ossification of fetal bones) to confirm position and presentation; not used in early pregnancy to avoid possibility of causing damage to fetus and mother.

   e. *Alpha-fetoprotein screening*: Maternal serum screens. Alpha-fetoprotein is glucoprotein produced by fetal yolk sac, GI tract, and liver. Test done between 15 and 18 weeks' gestation. Elevated AFP may be associated with neural tube defects, renal anomalies. Low AFP seen with chromosomal trisomies.

   f. *L/S ratio*: uses amniotic fluid to ascertain fetal lung maturity through measurement of presence and amounts of the lung surfactants lecithin and sphingomyelin. At 35–36 weeks, ratio is 2:1, indicative of mature levels; once ratio of 2:1 is achieved, newborn less likely to develop respiratory distress syndrome. Phosphatidylglycerol (PG) is found in amniotic fluid after 35 weeks. In conjunction with the L/S ratio, it contributes to increased reliability of fetal lung maturity testing. May be done in laboratory or by "shake" test.

   g. Fetal movement count: teach mother to count 2–3 times daily, 30–60 minutes each time, should feel 5–6 movements per counting time. Mother should notify care giver immediately of abrupt change or no movement.

   h. PUBS (percutaneous umbilical blood sampling): uses ultrasound to locate umbilical cord. Cord blood aspirated and tested. Used in second and third trimesters.

   i. Biophysical profile: a collection of data on fetal breathing movements, body movements, muscle tone, reactive heart rate, and amniotic fluid volume. A score of 0 to 2 is given in each category, and the summative number interpreted by the physician. Primary suggested use is to identify fetuses at risk for asphyxia.

B. Electronic Monitoring

   1. Nonstress test (NST) (see Table 3-2)

      a. Accelerations in heart rate accompany normal fetal movement

      b. In high-risk pregnancies, NST may be used to assess FHR on a frequent basis in order to ascertain fetal well-being.

      c. Noninvasive

26 Chapter 3

TABLE 3-2 Nonstress Test (NST)

Result	Interpretation	Significance
Reactive	2 or more accelerations of 15 beats/min lasting 15 sec or more in 20-min period (associated with each fetal movement)	High-risk pregnancy allowed to continue if twice weekly NSTs are reactive.
Nonreactive	No FHR acceleration, or accelerations less than 15 beats/min or lasting less than 15 sec through fetal movement	Need to attempt to clarify FHR pattern; implement CST and continue external monitoring.
Unsatisfactory	FHR pattern not able to be interpreted	Repeat NST or do CST.

TABLE 3-3 Contraction Stress Test (CST)

Result	Interpretation	Significance
Negative	3 contractions, 40–60 sec long, within 10-min period, no late decelerations	Fetus should tolerate labor if it occurs within 1 week.
Positive	Persistent/consistent late decelerations with more than 50% of contractions	Fetus at increased risk. May need additional testing, may try induction or cesarean birth.
Suspicious	Late decelerations in less than 50% of contractions	Repeat CST in 24 hr, or other fetal assessment tests.
Unsatisfactory	Inadequate pattern or poor tracing	Same as for suspicious.

    2. Contraction stress test (CST) (see Table 3-3)

        a. Based on principle that healthy fetus can withstand decreased oxygen during contraction, but compromised fetus cannot.

CLIENT TEACHING CHECKLIST

Instruct the client about the following potential medical emergencies during pregnancy:

- Vaginal bleeding
- Ruptured membranes
- Severe headache
- Visual disturbances
- Abdominal pain
- Epigastric pain
- Edema of face and hands

    b. Types
        1) nipple-stimulated CST: massage or rolling of one or both nipples to stimulate uterine activity and check effect on FHR.
        2) oxytocin challenge test (OCT): infusion of calibrated dose of IV oxytocin "piggybacked" to main IV line; controlled by infusion pump; amount infused increased every 15–20 minutes until three good uterine contractions are observed within 10-minute period.
        3) CST never done unless willing to deliver fetus.

■ EVALUATION

A. Maternal/fetal assessment data remain within acceptable limits; fetus maintains growth and development pattern appropriate to gestational age (evidenced by maternal weight gain, normal increments in fundal height, fetal activity level, other antepartal tests).
B. No complications of pregnancy are evident.
    1. Pregnant woman receives prenatal care (initial and subsequent visits).
    2. Maternal blood pressure, weight gain, and other lab test findings are within normal range.
C. Pregnant woman/family have received adequate educational instruction.
    1. Pregnant woman/family express understanding of childbirth experience and begin transition to role of parenting.
    2. Any necessary testing procedures carried out completely and correctly; client/fetus in stable condition.

■ COMPLICATIONS OF PREGNANCY

Pregnancy can be complicated by situations unique to childbearing (e.g., placental bleeding), or by longstanding conditions predating pregnancy and

TABLE 3-4 Common Discomforts during Pregnancy

Discomfort	Trimester	Intervention
Morning sickness	First	Eat dry carbohydrate in AM; avoid fried, odorous, and greasy foods; small meals rather than large.
Fatigue	First	Rest frequently, as needed.
Urinary frequency	First, end of third	Kegel exercises, perineal pad for leakage.
Heartburn	Second, third	Small meals, bland foods, antacids if ordered.
Constipation	Second, third	Sufficient fluids, foods high in roughage, regular bowel habits. No laxatives unless ordered, including mineral oil.
Hemorrhoids	Third	Avoid constipation; promote regular bowel habits.
Varicosities	Third	Avoid crossing legs and long periods of sitting or standing; rest with feet and hips elevated; avoid elastic garters and other constrictive clothing.
Backache	Third	Use good posture and body mechanics; low-heeled shoes; exercises to strengthen back muscles.
Insomnia	Third	Conscious relaxation; supportive pillows as needed; warm shower before retiring.
Leg cramps	Third	Flex toes toward knees for relief; ensure adequate calcium in diet.
Supine hypotensive syndrome	Third	Left side-lying position.

Vaginal discharge	Second	Correct personal hygiene, refer to physician. Do not douche.
Skin changes, dryness, itching	All	Interventions are symptomatic; cool baths, lotions, oils as indicated.

continuing into the childbearing process (e.g., age, socioeconomic status, cardiac problems); for common discomforts of pregnancy, see Table 3-4.

General Nursing Responsibilities

A. Teach danger signals of pregnancy early in prenatal period so that client is aware of what needs to be reported to health care provider on an immediate basis (see Table 3-5).
B. Be aware that early teaching allows the client to participate in the identification and reporting of symptoms that can indicate a problem in her pregnancy.
C. Early recognition and reporting of danger signals usually results in diminishing the risk and controlling the severity of maternal/fetal complications.
D. Interventions are specific for the individual risks.
E. Evaluation centers around whether or not the risk was controlled or eliminated, and how the maternal/fetal reaction was controlled.

First Trimester Bleeding Complications

Abortion

A. General information
   1. Loss of pregnancy before viability of fetus; may be spontaneous, therapeutic, or elective (for additional information on therapeutic and

TABLE 3-5   Danger Signals of Pregnancy

- Any bleeding from vagina
- Gush of fluid from vagina (clear, not urine)
- Regular contractions occurring before due date
- Severe headaches or changes in vision
- Epigastric pain
- Vomiting that persists and is severe
- Change in fetal activity patterns
- Temperature elevation, chills, or "sick" feeling indicative of infection
- Swelling in upper body, especially face and fingers

CLIENT TEACHING CHECKLIST

Encourage the client to report any vaginal bleeding or other fluid leakage.

DELEGATION TIP

Encourage client to be aware of fetal movement and to report decreased or lack of movement if longer than 6–8 hours.

elective abortions see Control of Fertility, page 609). (Clients may use term "miscarriage" for spontaneous abortion.)

2. Types
   a. Threatened abortion
      1) cervix closed
      2) some bleeding and contractions
      3) fetus not expelled
   b. Inevitable
      1) cervix open
      2) heavier bleeding and stronger contractions
      3) loss of fetus usually not avoidable
   c. Incomplete
      1) expulsion of fetus incomplete
      2) membranes or placenta retained
   d. Complete: all products of conception expelled
   e. Missed: fetus dies in uterus but is not expelled
   f. Habitual
      1) three pregnancies in a row culminating in spontaneous abortion
      2) may indicate need for investigation into underlying causes
B. Assessment findings
   1. Vaginal bleeding (observing carefully for accurate determination of amount, saving all perineal pads)
   2. Contractions, pelvic cramping, backache
   3. Lowered hemoglobin if blood loss significant
   4. Passage of fetus/tissue
C. Nursing interventions
   1. Save all tissue passed.
   2. Keep client at rest and teach reason for bed rest.
   3. Increase fluids PO or IV.
   4. Prepare client for surgical intervention (D&C or suction evacuation) if needed (see also Termination of Pregnancy).

5. Provide discharge teaching about limited activities and coitus after bleeding ceases.
6. Observe reaction of mother and others, provide emotional support, and give opportunity to express feelings of grief and loss.
7. Administer Rhogam if mother Rh negative.

Incompetent Cervical Os (Premature Dilation of Cervix)

A. General information: painless condition in which the cervix dilates without uterine contractions and allows passage of the fetus; usually the result of prior cervical trauma.
B. Medical management: may be treated surgically by cerclage (placement of fascia or artificial material to constrict the cervix in a "purse-string" manner). When client goes into labor, choice of removal of suture and vaginal delivery, or cesarean birth.
C. Assessment findings
   1. History of repeated, relatively painless abortions
   2. Early and progressive effacement and dilation of cervix, usually second trimester
   3. Bulging of membranes through cervical os
D. Nursing interventions
   1. Continue observation for contractions, rupture of membranes, and monitor fetal heart tones.
   2. Position client to minimize pressure on cervix.

Ectopic Pregnancy

A. General information
   1. Any gestation outside the uterine cavity
   2. Most frequent in the fallopian tubes, where the tissue is incapable of the growth needed to accommodate pregnancy, so rupture of the site usually occurs before 12 weeks.
   3. Any condition that diminishes the tubal lumen may predispose a woman to ectopic pregnancy
B. Assessment findings
   1. History of missed periods and symptoms of early pregnancy
   2. Abdominal pain, may be localized to one side
   3. Rigid, tender abdomen; sometimes abnormal pelvic mass
   4. Bleeding; if severe may lead to shock
   5. Low hemoglobin and hematocrit, rising white cell count
   6. HCG titers usually lower than in intrauterine pregnancy
C. Nursing interventions
   1. Prepare client for surgery.
   2. Institute measures to control/treat shock if hemorrhage severe; continue to monitor postoperatively.

3. Allow client to express feelings about loss of pregnancy and concerns about future pregnancies.

Hydatidiform Mole (Gestational Trophoblastic Disease)

A. General information
   1. Proliferation of trophoblasts; embryo dies. Unusual chromosomal patterns seen (either no genetic material in ovum, or 69 chromosomes). The chorionic villi change into a mass of clear, fluid-filled grapelike vessels.
   2. More common in women over 40.
   3. Cause essentially unknown.
B. Assessment findings
   1. Increased size of uterus disproportionate to length of pregnancy
   2. High levels of HCG with excessive nausea and vomiting
   3. Dark red to brownish vaginal bleeding after 12th week
   4. Anemia often accompanies bleeding
   5. Symptoms of preeclampsia before usual time of onset
   6. No fetal heart sounds or palpation of fetal parts
   7. Ultrasound shows no fetal skeleton
C. Nursing interventions
   1. Provide pre- and postoperative care for evacuation of uterus (usually suction curettage).
   2. Teach contraceptive use so that pregnancy is delayed for at least one year.
   3. Teach client need for follow-up lab work to detect rising HCG levels indicative of choriocarcinoma.
   4. Provide emotional support for loss of pregnancy.
   5. Teach about risk for future pregnancies, if indicated.

Second Trimester Bleeding Complications

There are few unique causes of bleeding in the second trimester. Bleeding may be a late manifestation of condition usually seen in first trimester, such as spontaneous abortion or incompetent cervical os.

Third Trimester Bleeding Complications

Placental problems are the most frequent cause of bleeding in the third trimester.

Placenta Previa

A. General information
   1. Low implantation of the placenta so that it overlays some or all of the internal cervical os. Complete previa requires cesarean delivery. Partial may deliver vaginally if fetus in vertex presentation.
   2. Cause uncertain, but uterine factors (poor vascularity, fibroid tumors, multiple pregnancies) may be involved.

3. Amount of cervical os involved classifies placenta previa as marginal, partial, or complete.
4. Often diagnosed prior to 30 weeks by sonogram. Many resolve or migrate before labor.

B. Assessment findings
   1. Bright red, painless vaginal bleeding after seventh month of pregnancy is cardinal indicator. Bleeding may be intermittent, in gushes, or continuous.
   2. Uterus remains soft.
   3. FHR usually stable unless maternal shock present.
   4. No vaginal exam by nurse, may result in severe bleed, if done by physician, double setup used.
   5. Diagnosis by sonography.

C. Nursing interventions
   1. Ensure complete bed rest.
   2. Maintain sterile conditions for any invasive procedures (including vaginal examination).
   3. Make provision for emergency cesarean birth (*double set-up procedure*).
   4. Continue to monitor maternal/fetal vital signs.
   5. Measure blood loss carefully.
   6. Assess uterine tone regularly.

Abruptio Placentae

A. General information
   1. Separation of placenta from part or all of normal implantation site, usually accompanied by pain
   2. Usually occurs after 20th week of pregnancy
   3. Increased risk of abruption with maternal hypertension, previous abruption, cigarette smoking, multiparity, history of abortions, cocaine use, abdominal trauma

B. Assessment findings
   1. Painful vaginal bleeding
   2. Tender, boardlike uterus (especially if concealed hemorrhage, then no vaginal bleeding)
   3. Fetal bradycardia and late decelerations, absent FHT in complete abruption
   4. Additional signs of shock

C. Nursing interventions
   1. Ensure bed rest.
   2. Check maternal/fetal vital signs frequently.
   3. Prepare for IV infusions of fluids/blood as indicated.
   4. Monitor urinary output.
   5. Anticipate coagulation problems (DIC).

6. Provide support to parents as outlook for fetus is poor.
7. Prepare for emergency surgery as indicated.

Hyperemesis Gravidarum

A. General information
   1. Excess nausea and vomiting of early pregnancy leads to dehydration and electrolyte disturbances, especially acidosis.
   2. Causes: possible severe reaction to HCG, not psychological, greater risk in conditions where HCG levels increased. HCG levels peak around 6 weeks after conception, plateau, then begin to decline after the 12th week. Symptoms often improve later in pregnancy but may last entire time.
B. Assessment findings
   1. Nausea and vomiting, progressing to retching between meals
   2. Weight loss
C. Nursing interventions
   1. Begin NPO and IV fluid and electrolyte replacement. (Correction of F&E balance will decrease nausea, NPO will rest the stomach.)
   2. Monitor I&O.
   3. Gradually reintroduce PO intake, monitor amounts taken and retained.
   4. Monitor TPN and central line placement if unable to eat.
   5. Provide mouth care.
   6. Offer emotional support—very demoralizing and depressing to client.
   7. Refer to home health as appropriate for continued IV or TPN therapy.

Pregnancy-Induced Hypertension

General Information

A. Refers to condition unique to pregnancy where vasospastic hypertension is accompanied by proteinuria and edema; maternal or fetal condition may be compromised.
   1. Probable cause: gradual loss of normal pregnancy-related response to angiotensin II
   2. May also be related to decreased production of some vasodilating prostaglandins
B. Onset after 20th week of pregnancy, may appear in labor or up to 48 hours postpartum.
C. Characterized by widespread vasospasm.
D. Cause essentially unknown, but incidence is high in primigravidas, multiple pregnancies, maternal age under 17 or over 35, hydatidiform mole, poor nutrition, essential hypertension; familial tendency.
E. Occurs in 5-7% of all pregnant women.

F. Clinical classification of hypertensive disorders in pregnancy.
  1. Pregnancy-induced hypertension (PIH)
      a. Preeclampsia—mild or severe
      b. Eclampsia
  2. Chronic hypertension
  3. Chronic hypertension with superimposed PIH
G. Classic triad of symptoms includes edema/weight gain, hypertension, and proteinuria. Eclampsia includes convulsions and coma.
H. Possible life-threatening complication: HELLP syndrome (*h*emolysis, *e*levated *l*iver enzymes, *l*owered *p*latelets).
I. Only known cure is delivery.

Mild Preeclampsia

A. Assessment findings
  1. Appearance of symptoms between 20th and 24th week of pregnancy
  2. Blood pressure of 140/90 or $+30$ systolic/$+15$ mmHg diastolic on two consecutive occasions at least 6 hours apart
  3. Sudden weight gain ($+3$ lb/month in second trimester; $+1$ lb/week in third trimester; or $+4.5$ lb/week at any time)
  4. Slight generalized edema, especially of hands and face
  5. Proteinuria of 300 mg/liter in a 24-hour specimen ($+1$ in 1 specimen)
B. Nursing interventions
  1. Promote bed rest as long as signs of edema or proteinuria are minimal, preferably side-lying.
  2. Provide well-balanced diet with adequate protein and roughage, no Na^+ restriction.
  3. Explain need for close follow-up, weekly or twice-weekly visits to physician.

Severe Preeclampsia

A. Assessment findings
  1. Headaches, epigastric pain, nausea and vomiting, visual disturbances, irritability
  2. Blood pressure of 150–160/100–110
  3. Increased edema and weight gain
  4. Proteinuria (5 g/24 hours) ($4+$) oliguria
  5. Hyperreflexia of $4+$, possibly with clonus
B. Medical management: magnesium sulfate
  1. Magnesium sulfate acts upon the myoneural junction, diminishing neuromuscular transmission.

2. It promotes maternal vasodilation, better tissue perfusion, and has anticonvulsant effect.
3. Nursing responsibilities
   a. Monitor client's respirations, blood pressure, and reflexes, as well as urinary output frequently.
   b. Administer medications either IV or IM.
4. Antidote for excess levels of magnesium sulfate is calcium gluconate or calcium chloride.

C. Nursing interventions
   1. Promote complete bed rest, side-lying.
   2. Carefully monitor maternal/fetal vital signs.
   3. Monitor I&O, results of laboratory tests.
   4. Take daily weights.
   5. Do daily fundoscopic examination.
   6. Institute seizure precautions.
      a. Restrict visitors.
      b. Minimize all stimuli.
      c. Monitor for hyperreflexia.
      d. Administer sedatives as ordered.
   7. Instruct client about appropriate diet.
   8. Continue to monitor 24–48 hours postdelivery.
   9. Administer medications as ordered; vasodilator of choice usually hydralazine (Apresoline).

Eclampsia

A. Medical management (see Severe Preeclampsia).
B. Assessment findings
   1. Increased hypertension precedes convulsion followed by hypotension and collapse.
   2. Coma may ensue.
   3. Labor may begin, putting fetus in great jeopardy.
   4. Convulsion may recur.
C. Nursing interventions
   1. Minimize all stimuli.
      a. Darken room.
      b. Limit visitors.
      c. Use padded bedsides and bed rails.
   2. Check vital signs and lab values frequently.
   3. Seizure precautions: airway, oxygen, and suction equipment should be available at bedside.
   4. Administer medications as ordered.
   5. Prepare for C-section when seizures stabilized.
   6. Continue observations 24–48 hours postpartum.

■ PRE- AND COEXISTING DISEASES OF PREGNANCY
Cardiac Conditions
General Information
A. May be the result of congenital heart disease or the sequelae of rheumatic fever/heart disease.
B. May affect pregnancy, but are definitely affected by pregnancy.
C. Classification
   1. Class 1: no limitation of activity
   2. Class 2: slight limitation of activity
   3. Class 3: considerable limitation of activity
   4. Class 4: symptoms present even at rest

Prenatal Period
A. Assessment findings
   1. Evidence of cardiac decompensation especially when blood volume peaks (weeks 28-32)
   2. Cough and dyspnea
   3. Edema
   4. Heart murmurs
   5. Palpitations
   6. Rales
B. Nursing interventions
   1. Promote frequent rest periods and adequate sleep, decreased stress.
   2. Teach client to recognize and report signs of infection, importance of prophylactic antibiotics.
   3. Compare vital signs to baseline and normal values expected during pregnancy.
   4. Instruct in diet to limit weight gain to 15 lb., low Na^+.
   5. Explain rationale for anticoagulant therapy (heparin used in pregnancy) if ordered.
   6. Teach danger signals for individual client.

Intrapartal Period
A. Labor increases risk of congestive heart failure: milking effect of contractions and delivery increases blood volume to heart.
B. Nursing interventions
   1. Monitor maternal EKG and FHT continuously.
   2. Explain to client that vaginal delivery is preferred over C-section.
   3. Monitor client's response to stress of labor and watch for signs of decompensation.
   4. Administer oxygen and pain medication as ordered, epidural preferable.

5. Position client in side-lying/low semi-Fowler's position.
6. Provide calm atmosphere.
7. Encourage "open-glottal" pushing during second stage of labor, forceps or vacuum extractor used to minimize pushing.

Postpartal Period

A. Nursing interventions
   1. Monitor vital signs, any bleeding, strict I&O, lab test values, daily weight, rest and diet.
   2. Promote bed rest in appropriate position (see Intrapartal Period above).
   3. Assist with activities of daily living (ADL) as needed.
   4. Prevent infection.
   5. Facilitate nonstressful mother/baby interactions.
   6. Help mother plan for rest and activity patterns at home, as well as household help if indicated.

Endocrine Conditions

Diabetes Mellitus

A. General information
   1. Chronic disease caused by improper metabolic interaction of carbohydrates, fats, proteins, and insulin.
   2. Interaction of pregnancy and diabetes may cause serious complications of pregnancy.
   3. Classifications of diabetes mellitus
      a. Type I, insulin-dependent diabetes mellitus, usually appears before age 30
      b. Type II, noninsulin-dependent, onset usually after age 30
      c. Gestational diabetes, onset occurs during pregnancy
   4. Significance of diabetes in pregnancy
      a. Interaction of estrogen, progesterone, HCS/HPL, and cortisol raise maternal resistance to insulin (ability to use glucose at the cellular level).
      b. If the pancreas cannot respond by producing additional insulin, excess glucose moves across placenta to fetus, where fetal insulin metabolizes it, and acts as growth hormone, promoting macrosomia.
      c. Maternal insulin levels need to be carefully monitored during pregnancy to avoid widely fluctuating levels of blood glucose.
      d. Dose may drop during first trimester, then rise during second and third trimesters.
      e. Higher incidence of fetal anomalies and neonatal hypoglycemia (good control minimizes).

B. Assessment findings: signs of hyperglycemia
  1. Polyuria
  2. Polydipsia
  3. Weight loss
  4. Polyphagia
  5. Elevated glucose levels in blood and urine. Urine tests for elevated blood glucose less reliable in pregnancy. Blood tests (more accurate) used as follows
    a. 1-hour glucose tolerance test: usually done for screening on all pregnant women 24–28 weeks pregnant.
    b. 3-hour glucose tolerance test: used where results from 1 hour GTT > 140 mg/dl.
    c. HbA_{1c}: glycosylated hemoglobin; reflects past 4–12-week blood levels of serum glucose.
C. Nursing interventions
  1. Teach client the effects and interactions of diabetes and pregnancy and signs of hyper- and hypoglycemia.
  2. Teach client how to control diabetes in pregnancy, advise of changes that need to be made in nutrition and activity patterns to promote normal glucose levels and prevent complications.
  3. Advise client of increased risk of infection and how to avoid it.
  4. Observe and report any signs of preeclampsia.
  5. Monitor fetal status throughout pregnancy.
  6. Assess status of mother and baby frequently
    a. Monitor carefully fluids, calories, glucose, and insulin during labor and delivery.
    b. Continue careful observation in postdelivery period.

Renal Conditions

Urinary Tract Infections (UTI)

A. General information
  1. Affect 10% of all pregnant women.
  2. Dilated, flaccid, and displaced ureters are a frequent site.
  3. *E. coli* is the usual cause.
  4. May cause premature labor if severe, untreated, or pyelonephritis develops.
B. Assessment findings
  1. Frequency and urgency of urination
  2. Suprapubic pain
  3. Flank pain (if kidney involved)
  4. Hematuria
  5. Pyuria
  6. Fever and chills

C. Nursing interventions
1. Encourage high fluid intake.
2. Provide warm baths to relieve discomfort and promote perineal hygiene.
3. Administer and monitor intake of prescribed medications (antibiotics, urinary analgesics).
4. Stress good bladder-emptying schedule.
5. Monitor for signs of premature labor from severe or untreated infection.

Other Infections

A. General information
1. Pregnancy is not a prevention against pre- or coexisting infections.
2. *T*oxoplasmosis, *o*ther infections, *r*ubella, *c*ytomegalovirus, and *h*erpes (*TORCH infections*) are especially devastating to the fetus, causing abortions, malformations, and even fetal death.
3. Rubella titer is assessed during early prenatal visit. If mother is deficient in rubella antibodies (titer less than 1.0), rubella virus vaccine is recommended in immediate postpartum period.
B. General nursing interventions
1. Instruct the pregnant woman in signs and symptoms that indicate infection, especially fever, chills, sore throat, localized pain, or rash.
2. Caution pregnant women to avoid obviously infected persons and other sources of infection, as danger exists for the fetus in all maternal infections.
3. May affect delivery options.

AIDS and Pregnancy

A. General information
1. Transmission of the human immunodeficiency virus authenticated through blood, semen, vaginal secretions, and breast milk.
2. Can be transmitted from mother to fetus during pregnancy.
3. Cesarean delivery will not avert mother-to-fetus transmission.
4. Breastfeeding not currently recommended for seropositive mothers.
5. Increase in prematurity, premature rupture of membranes, low birth weight, and coexistent STDs.
6. Pregnancy-altered immune states may result in the acceleration of opportunistic diseases, such as *Candida albicans*, herpes, and toxoplasmosis.
7. Treatment of the mother with AZT during pregnancy decreases the risk of transmission of the virus to the fetus.
B. Nursing implications
1. Thorough review of history and any physical symptoms.
2. Close attention to lab studies, especially CBC, leukocyte count, T-cell count, and urinalysis indicated.
3. Strict attention to universal precautions as appropriate.

4. Protective coverings in delivery room.
5. Wear gloves to handle all infants until they are bathed.
6. Suction newborn with bulb or wall suction devices only.
7. Special assessments: respiratory, neurologic, psychosocial.

Other Conditions of Risk in Pregnancy

Adolescence

A. General information
   1. Pregnancy is a condition of both physical and psychologic risk.
   2. Adolescent is frequently undernourished and not yet completely matured either physically or psychosocially.
   3. Adolescent is uniquely unsuited for the stresses of pregnancy.
   4. Frequency of serious complications increases in adolescent pregnancy, particularly toxemia and low-birth-weight infants.
B. Nursing interventions
   1. Encourage adequate prenatal care.
   2. Provide health teaching to prepare for pregnancy, labor and delivery, and motherhood.
   3. Provide nutritional counseling.
   4. Teach coping skills for labor and delivery.
   5. Teach child care skills.

Disseminated Intravascular Coagulation (DIC)

A. General information
   1. Also known as *consumptive coagulopathy*
   2. A diffuse, pathologic form of clotting, secondary to underlying disease/pathology.
   3. Occurs in critical maternity problems such as abruptio placenta, dead fetus syndrome, amniotic fluid embolism, preeclampsia/eclampsia, hydatidiform mole, and hemorrhagic shock
   4. Mechanism
      a. Precoagulant substances released in the blood trigger microthrombosis in peripheral vessels and paradoxical consumption of circulating clotting factors.
      b. Fibrin-split products accumulate, further interfering with the clotting process.
      c. Platelet and fibrinogen levels drop.
B. Assessment findings
   1. Bleeding may range from massive, unanticipated blood loss to localized bleeding (purpura and petechiae)
   2. Presence of special maternity problems
   3. Prolonged prothrombin and partial thromboplastin times
C. Nursing interventions
   1. Assist with medical management of underlying condition.

2. Administer blood component therapy (white blood cells, packed cells, fresh frozen plasma, cryoprecipitate) as ordered.
3. Observe for signs of insidious bleeding (oozing IV site, petechiae, lowered hematocrit).
4. Institute nursing measures for severe bleeding/shock if needed.
5. Provide emotional support to client and family as needed.

Anemia

A. General information
   1. Low red cell count may be underlying condition
   2. May or may not be exacerbated by physiologic hemodilution of pregnancy
   3. Most common medical disorder of pregnancy
B. Assessment findings
   1. Client is pale, tired, short of breath, dizzy.
   2. Hgb is less than 11 g/dl; hct less than 37%.
C. Nursing interventions
   1. Encourage intake of foods with high iron content.
   2. Monitor iron supplementation.
   3. Teach sequelae of iron ingestion.
   4. Assess need for parenteral iron.

Prenatal Substance Abuse

A. General information
   1. Incidence: probably underestimated in our society.
   2. Morbidity/mortality: related to chemical used, timing, and route of administration.
B. Assessment findings
   1. Alcohol
      a. Elevates the mood, depresses the central nervous system
      b. Affects every other system in the body of the mother
      c. Displaces other nutritional food intake
      d. Greatest risk from high blood alcohol levels
      e. No safe level of maternal alcohol use in pregnancy has been established
      f. Fetus may display IUGR (intrauterine growth retardation), CNS dysfunction, and craniofacial abnormalities (fetal alcohol syndrome).
   2. Cocaine
      a. Powerful stimulant; very addictive
      b. Causes vasoconstriction, elevated BP, tachycardia
      c. May precipitate seizures
      d. Affects ability to transport O_2 into the blood
      e. May cause spontaneous abortion, fetal malformation, placenta abruptio, neural tube defects

   f. Newborn may display irritability, hypertonicity, poor feeding patterns, increased risk of SIDS

 3. Opiates

   a. Produce analgesia, euphoria, respiratory depression

   b. If used IV, foreign substance contamination may cause pulmonary emboli or infections

   c. If used IV, places mother at greater risk of contracting HIV, then passing it on to fetus

   d. Newborns experience withdrawal within 24–72 hours after delivery

   e. High-pitched cry, restlessness, poor feeding seen in the newborn

 4. Other chemicals

   a. May include tranquilizers, prescription medications, paint thinners, other aerosols, etc.

   b. Major danger is overdose, with accompanying cardiac/respiratory arrest

C. Nursing interventions

 1. Treatment during pregnancy may include in- or outpatient care. Alcoholics Anonymous-based programs are widely utilized.

 2. Treatment may include family therapy.

 3. Efforts to treat the chemical abuse/dependency should be maximized during pregnancy. Withdrawal is best accomplished with competent, professional help.

REVIEW QUESTIONS

1. A 22-year-old has missed two of her regular menstrual periods. Her doctor confirms an early, intrauterine pregnancy. This is her first pregnancy. To determine her expected due date, which of the following assessments is most important?

 1. Dates of first menstrual period.

 2. Date of last intercourse.

 3. Dates of last normal menstrual period.

 4. Age at menarche.

2. A 24-year-old woman is pregnant with her first baby. During her seventh month, she complains of backache. The nurse teaches her to

 1. sleep on a soft mattress.

 2. walk barefoot at least once/day.

 3. perform Kegel exercises once/day.

 4. wear low-heeled shoes.

3. A woman is hospitalized for the treatment of severe preeclampsia. Which of the following represents an unusual finding for this condition?
   1. Convulsions.
   2. Blood pressure 160/100.
   3. Proteinuria 3+.
   4. Generalized edema.

4. A woman is admitted with severe preeclampsia. What type of room should the nurse select for this woman?
   1. A room next to the elevator.
   2. The room farthest from the nursing station.
   3. The quietest room on the floor.
   4. The labor suite.

5. The action of hormones during pregnancy affects the body by
   1. raising resistance to insulin.
   2. blocking the release of insulin from the pancreas.
   3. preventing the liver from metabolizing glycogen.
   4. enhancing the conversion of food to glucose.

6. A 28-year-old has had diabetes mellitus since she was an adolescent. She is 8 weeks pregnant. Hyperglycemia during her first trimester will have what effect on the fetus?
   1. Hyperinsulinemia.
   2. Excessive fetal size.
   3. Malformed organs.
   4. Abnormal positioning.

7. The nurse is caring for a young diabetic woman who is in her first trimester of pregnancy. As the pregnancy continues the nurse should anticipate which change in her medication needs?
   1. A decrease in the need for short-acting insulins.
   2. A steady increase in insulin requirements.
   3. Oral hypoglycemic drugs will be given several times daily.
   4. The variable pattern of insulin absorption throughout the pregnancy requires constant close adjustment.

8. A glycosylated hemoglobin level is ordered for a pregnant diabetic because it
   1. is the most accurate method of determining present insulin levels.
   2. will predict how well the pancreas can respond to the stress of pregnancy.

3. indicates mean glucose level over a 1- to 3-month period.

4. gives diagnostic information related to the peripheral effects of diabetes.

9. A 25-year-old has been coming to the prenatal clinic on a regular basis. She is 5 months pregnant. She suffered from morning sickness early in her pregnancy and is now concerned because the vomiting has continued and she is feeling weak and exhausted. Diagnosed as having hyperemesis gravidarum, she is hospitalized and parenteral fluid therapy is started. She has vomited twice within the last hour. The immediate nursing intervention would be to

1. assist her with mouth care.

2. notify the physician.

3. change the IV infusion to Ringer's lactate.

4. warm her tray and serve it to her again.

10. A woman in her seventh month of pregnancy has a hemoglobin of 10.5 g. The nurse teaches the woman about proper nutrition during pregnancy. Which statement made by the client indicates to the nurse that teaching was effective?

1. "I eat liver once a week."

2. "I have an orange for breakfast."

3. "I eat six small meals a day."

4. "I have a green leafy vegetable occasionally."

11. A couple recently arrived in the United States from East Asia. The man brings his wife to the hospital in late labor; his mother and the woman's sister are also present. As the nurse directs the man to the dressing room to change into a scrub suit, his wife anxiously states, "No, he can't come with me. Get my sister and mother-in-law!" The nurse's best response is,

1. "I'm sorry, but our hospital only allows the father into the delivery."

2. "I'll ask the doctor if that's OK."

3. "When I talk to your husband, I'm sure he'll want to be with you."

4. "That's fine. I'll show your husband the waiting area."

12. During an initial prenatal visit, a woman states that her last menstrual period began on November 21; she also reports some vaginal bleeding about December 19. The nurse would calculate that this client's expected date of birth (EDB) would be

1. July 21.

2. August 28.

3. September 26.

4. October 1.

13. A 24-year-old woman comes to the clinic because she thinks she is pregnant. Which of the following is a probable sign of pregnancy that the nurse would expect this client to have?

    1. Fetal heart tones.

    2. Nausea and vomiting.

    3. Amenorrhea.

    4. Chadwick's sign.

14. A married 25-year-old housewife is 6 weeks' gestation and is being seen for her first prenatal visit. In relation to normal maternal acceptance of pregnancy, the nurse would expect that the client feels

    1. some ambivalence now that the pregnancy is confirmed.

    2. overwhelmed by the thought of future changes.

    3. much happiness and enjoyment in the event.

    4. detached from the event until physical changes occur.

15. A woman is entering the 20th week of pregnancy. Which normal change would the nurse expect to find on assessment?

    1. Fundus just below diaphragm.

    2. Pigment changes in skin.

    3. Complaints of frequent urination.

    4. Blood pressure returning to prepregnancy level.

16. A primigravida in the first trimester is blood type A+, rubella negative, hemoglobin 12 g, hematocrit 36%. During her second prenatal visit she complains of being very tired, experiencing frequent urination, and a white vaginal discharge; she also states that her nausea and occasional vomiting persist. Based on these findings, the nurse would select which of the following nursing diagnoses?

    1. Activity intolerance related to nutritional deprivation.

    2. Impaired urinary elimination related to a possible infection.

    3. Risk for injury related to hematologic incompatibility.

    4. Alteration in physiologic responses related to pregnancy.

17. A young woman had her pregnancy confirmed and has completed her first prenatal visit. Considering that all data were found to be within normal limits, the nurse would plan that the next visit should be in

    1. one week.

    2. two weeks.

    3. one month.

    4. two months.

18. Which statement by a pregnant client would indicate to the nurse that diet teaching has been effective?

　1. "The most important time to take my iron pills is during the early weeks when the baby is forming."

　2. "I don't like milk, but I'll increase my intake of cheese and yogurt."

　3. "I'll be very careful about using salt while I'm pregnant."

　4. "Because I'm overweight to begin with, I can continue my weight loss diet."

19. A woman, age 40, gravida 3 para 2, is 8 weeks pregnant. She is a full-time office manager and states she "usually unwinds with a few glasses of wine" with dinner, smokes about five cigarettes a day, and was "surprised" by this pregnancy. After the assessment, which of the following would the nurse select as the priority nursing diagnosis?

　1. Risk for an impaired bonding related to an unplanned pregnancy.

　2. Risk for injury to the fetus related to advanced age.

　3. Ineffective individual coping related to low self-esteem.

　4. Deficient knowledge related to effects of substance abuse.

20. A young couple has just completed a preconception visit in the maternity clinic. Before leaving, the woman asks the nurse why she was instructed not to take any over-the-counter medications. The nurse should reply

　1. "Research has found that many of these drugs have been linked to problems with getting pregnant."

　2. "At conception, and in the first trimester, these drugs can be as dangerous to the fetus as prescription drugs."

　3. "You should only take drugs that the physician has ordered during pregnancy."

　4. "Any drug is dangerous at this time; later on in pregnancy it won't matter."

21. The pregnant couple asks the nurse what is the purpose of prepared childbirth classes. The nurse's best response would be

　1. "The main goal of most types of childbirth classes is to provide information that will help eliminate fear and anxiety."

　2. "The desired goal is childbirth without the use of analgesics."

　3. "These classes help to reduce the pain of childbirth by exercise and relaxation methods."

　4. "The primary aim is to keep you and your baby healthy during pregnancy and after!"

22. A woman in her 38th week of pregnancy is to have an amniocentesis to evaluate fetal maturity. The L/S (lecithin/sphingomyelin) ratio is 2:1. The nurse knows that this finding indicates

    1. fetal lung maturity.

    2. that labor can be induced.

    3. the fetus is not viable.

    4. a nonstress test is indicated.

23. A woman is having a contraction stress test (CST) in her last month of pregnancy. When assessing the fetal monitor strip, the nurse notices that with most of the contractions, the fetal heart rate uniformly slows at mid-contraction and then returns to baseline about 20 seconds after the contraction is over. The nurse would interpret the test result to be

    1. negative: normal.

    2. reactive negative.

    3. positive: abnormal.

    4. unsatisfactory.

24. A woman, 36 weeks' gestation, is having a CST with an oxytocin IV infusion pump. After two contractions, the uterus stays contracted. The best initial action of the nurse is to

    1. help the client turn on her left side.

    2. turn off the infusion pump.

    3. wait 3 minutes for the uterus to relax.

    4. administer prn terbutaline sulfate (Brethine).

25. A pregnant woman, in the first trimester, is to have a transabdominal ultrasound. The nurse would include which of the following instructions?

    1. Nothing by mouth (NPO) from 6:00 A.M. the morning of the test.

    2. Drink one to two quarts of water and do not urinate before the test.

    3. Come to the clinic first for injection of the contrast dye.

    4. No special instructions are needed for this test.

26. A woman who is pregnant for the first time calls the clinic to say she is bleeding. To obtain important information, the nurse should next ask,

    1. "When did you last feel the baby move?"

    2. "How long have you been pregnant?"

    3. "When was your pregnancy test done?"

    4. "Are you having any uterine cramping?"

27. A woman is hospitalized with a possible ectopic pregnancy. In addition to the classic symptoms of abdominal pain, amenorrhea, and abnormal vaginal bleeding, the nurse knows that which of the following factors in the woman's history may be associated with this condition?

   1. Multiparity.
   2. Age under 20.
   3. Pelvic inflammatory disease (PID).
   4. Habitual spontaneous abortions.

28. A woman is being discharged after treatment for a hydatidiform mole. The nurse should include which of the following in the discharge teaching plan?

   1. Do not become pregnant for at least one year.
   2. Have blood pressure checked weekly for 6 months.
   3. RhoGAM must be received with next pregnancy and delivery.
   4. An amniocentesis can detect a recurrence of this disorder in the future.

29. A woman, 40 weeks' gestation, is admitted to the labor and delivery unit with possible placenta previa. On the admission assessment, the nurse would expect to find

   1. signs of a Couvelaire uterus.
   2. severe lower abdominal pain.
   3. painless vaginal bleeding.
   4. a board-like abdomen.

30. A woman, 30 weeks' gestation, is being discharged to home care with a diagnosis of placenta previa. The nurse knows that the client understands her care at home when the client states,

   1. "As I get closer to my due date I will have to remain in bed."
   2. "I can continue with my office job because it's mostly sitting."
   3. "My husband won't be too happy with this 'no sex' order."
   4. "I'm disappointed that I will need a cesarean section."

31. A teenage client, 38 weeks' gestation, is admitted with a diagnosis of pregnancy-induced hypertension (PIH). Data include: blood pressure 160/100, generalized edema, weight gain of 10 pounds in last 2 weeks, and proteinuria of +3; the client is also complaining of a headache and nausea. In planning care for this client, the nurse would set the following priority goal. The client will

   1. demonstrate a decreased blood pressure within 48 hours.
   2. not experience a seizure prior to delivery.

3. maintain a strict diet prior to delivery.

4. comply with medical and nutritional regimen.

32. A woman, 32 weeks' gestation, has developed mild PIH. The nurse evaluates that the client understands her treatment regimen when the client states,

1. "It is most important not to miss any of my blood pressure medication."

2. "I will watch my diet restrictions very carefully."

3. "I will spend most of my time in bed, on my left side."

4. "I'm happy that this only happens during a first pregnancy."

33. A pregnant client with class 3 cardiac disease is seen during an initial prenatal visit. The nurse selects which of the following priority nursing diagnoses?

1. Knowledge deficit related to self-care during pregnancy.

2. Fear; client and family, related to pregnancy outcome.

3. Alteration in nutrition related to sodium-restricted diet.

4. Activity intolerance related to compromised cardiac status.

34. The nurse includes the importance of self-monitoring of glucose in the care plan for a diabetic client planning a pregnancy. The goal of this monitoring is to prevent

1. congenital malformations in the fetus.

2. maternal vasculopathy.

3. accelerated growth of the fetus.

4. delayed maturation of fetal lungs.

35. After a prenatal class on healthy behaviors during pregnancy, the nurse can evaluate that learning has occurred when a client states,

1. "Alcohol in the first trimester of pregnancy is very dangerous, later it's OK."

2. "Drinking alcohol during pregnancy is the most preventable cause of mental retardation."

3. "Alcohol is bad during pregnancy, but a little with breastfeeding helps with let-down."

4. "Problems for the baby usually only occur with heavy drinking of alcohol."

ANSWERS AND RATIONALES

1. 3. The dates of the last menstrual period, especially the first day of that period, will be used in applying Nagele's rule to determine the estimated date of delivery.

2. 4. A frequent cause of backache in the third trimester of pregnancy is the combined effect of relaxation of the sacroiliac joints and the change in the center of gravity of the pregnant woman due to the enlarging uterus. Wearing low-heeled shoes, especially when on her feet for extended periods of time, will help to minimize this discomfort.

3. 1. Convulsions are associated with an eclamptic condition.

4. 3. A quiet room in which stimuli are minimized and controlled is essential to the nursing care of the severely preeclamptic client.

5. 1. Hormonal influences during pregnancy cause a resistance to insulin utilization at the cellular level. It allows sufficient glucose for placental transport to the fetus, and also prevents the blood sugar in the nondiabetic client from falling to dangerous levels. In the diabetic client, it requires increases in her insulin doses.

6. 3. Major congenital malformations are noted in the insulin-dependent diabetic mother with poor metabolic control.

7. 2. During the first trimester of pregnancy, there is little change in insulin requirements. In the second trimester, gradually increasing amounts of insulin are needed, with the insulin dose doubling by the end of pregnancy.

8. 3. Glycosylated hemoglobin measurements can be used to assess prior glycemic control, giving the average over the past 1 to 3 months.

9. 1. Frequent vomiting irritates the oral mucosa and leaves the mouth very dry and foul tasting. The first nursing action should be aimed at relieving irritation and drying of the mouth by providing mouth care.

10. 1. Liver contains more iron than any other food source.

11. 4. Within the traditional East Asian family, roles are clearly defined. One consideration is the East Asian husband's lack of involvement during pregnancy and birth; this is a mutually agreeable separation of men's and women's roles.

12. 2. If a woman has a menstrual period every 28 days and was not taking oral contraceptives, Nägele's rule may be a fairly accurate determiner of her predicted birth date. To use this method, begin with the first day of the last menstrual period, subtract 3 months, and add 7 days.

13. 4. Probable signs of pregnancy are the result of physiologic changes in the pelvic organs and hormonal influences; for example, the mucous membranes of the vulva, vagina, and cervix become bluish (Chadwick's sign) as a result of hyperemia and proliferation of cells.

14. 1. During the first trimester of pregnancy, women normally experience ambivalence about being pregnant. It is estimated that around 80% of

women initially reject the idea of pregnancy; even women who planned pregnancy may respond at first with surprise and shock.

15. 2. From 20-24 weeks' gestation, pigment changes in skin may occur from actions of hormones. These include the linea nigra, melasma on the face, and striae gravidarum (stretch marks).

16. 4. All of the data stated are within the normal expected range for a first trimester pregnancy. These factors are related to hormonal changes and the growing uterus.

17. 3. In a low-risk pregnancy, the recommended frequency of prenatal visits is: every 4 weeks for the first 28 weeks, every 2 weeks until the 36th week, then every week until birth.

18. 2. To meet increased calcium needs, pregnant women need to increase their intake of dairy products or consider a calcium supplement that provides 600 mg of calcium per day; it is not necessary to drink milk.

19. 4. Evidence exists that smoking, consuming alcohol, or using social drugs during pregnancy may be harmful to the fetus.

20. 2. It is best to avoid any medication when planning a pregnancy and during the first trimester; the greatest potential for gross abnormalities in the fetus occurs during the first trimester, when fetal organs are first developing. The greatest danger extends from day 31 after the last menstrual period to day 71.

21. 1. All programs in prepared childbirth have some similarities; all have an educational component to help eliminate fear.

22. 1. Lecithin and sphingomyelin are phospholipids produced by the type II alveolar cells. The L/S ratio increases with gestation and a ratio of 2:1 indicates lung maturity.

23. 3. The CST subjects the fetus to uterine contractions that compress the arteries supplying the placenta, thus reducing placental blood flow and the flow of oxygen to the fetus; the fetus with minimal metabolic reserve will have late decelerations where the fetal heart rate does not return to the baseline until the contraction ends. Fetal compromise is therefore suggested.

24. 2. When IV oxytocin is being used to stimulate uterine contractions in a contraction stress test, the oxytocin infusion is stopped if contractions occur more often than every 2 minutes or last longer than 60 seconds, if uterine tetany (remains contracted) takes place, or if continued fetal heart rate decelerations are noted.

25. 2. To obtain clearer images during the first trimester, women are required to drink 1 to 2 quarts of clear fluid to fill the urinary bladder and thereby

push the uterus higher into the abdomen where it can be more accurately scanned.

26. 2. When a pregnant woman is bleeding vaginally, the nurse should first ask her how many weeks or months pregnant she is; management of bleeding differs in an early pregnancy contrasted with bleeding in late pregnancy. Additional information would include if tissue amniotic fluid was discharged and what other symptoms, such as cramps or pain, are present.

27. 3. The incidence of ectopic pregnancy in the United States has increased by a factor of 4.9 during recent years. This is attributed primarily to the growing number of women of childbearing age who experience PID and endometriosis, who use intrauterine devices, or who have had tubal surgery.

28. 1. The follow-up protocol of critical importance after a molar pregnancy is the assessment of serum chorionic gonadotropin (HCG); HCG is considered a highly specific tumor marker for gestational trophoblastic disease (GTD). The HCG levels are assayed at intervals for 1 year; a rise or plateau necessitates further diagnostic assessment and usually treatment. Pregnancy would obscure the evidence of choriocarcinoma by the normal secretion of HCG.

29. 3. Placenta previa, when the placenta is implanted in the lower uterine segment, often is characterized by the sudden onset of bright red bleeding in the third trimester. Usually this bleeding is painless and may or may not be accompanied by contractions.

30. 3. In placenta previa, any sexual arousal is contraindicated because it can cause the release of oxytocin, which can cause the cervix to pull away from the low-lying placenta; this results in bleeding and potential jeopardy to the fetus.

31. 2. Preeclampsia may progress to eclampsia, the convulsive phase of PIH. Symptoms that herald the progression include headache, visual disturbances, epigastric pain, nausea or vomiting, hyperreflexia, and oliguria; classical signs of PIH also intensify.

32. 3. Modified bed rest in the left lateral position may be advised for the client with mild PIH. This position improves venous return and placental and renal perfusion; urine output increases, and blood pressure may stabilize or decrease.

33. 4. Once pregnancy is established, the focus of management is on minimizing any extra cardiac demands on the pregnant woman. In class 3 cardiac disease, the client experiences fatigue, palpitation, dyspnea, or angina when she undertakes less than ordinary activity. Physical activity is markedly restricted; this includes bed rest throughout the pregnancy.

34. 1. There is increasing evidence that the degree of control for an insulin-dependent diabetic woman prior to conception greatly affects the fetal outcome. Studies find that poor maternal glucose control underlies the incidence of congenital malformations in the infants of diabetic mothers.

35. 2. Prenatal alcohol exposure is a preventable cause of birth defects and neurodevelopmental deficits; it is the leading most preventable cause of mental retardation.

4

Labor and Delivery

■ OVERVIEW

Five Factors of Labor (Five Ps)

Passenger

The size, presentation, and position of the fetus.

A. Fetal head (Figure 4-1)
   1. Usually the largest part of the baby; it has profound effect on birthing process.
   2. Bones of skull are joined by membranous sutures, which allow for overlapping or "molding" of cranial bones during birth process.
   3. *Anterior* and *posterior fontanels* are the points of intersection for the sutures and are important landmarks.
      a. Anterior fontanel is larger, diamond-shaped, and closes about 18 months of age.
      b. Posterior fontanel is smaller, triangular, and usually closes about 3 months of age.
   4. Fontanels are used as landmarks for internal examinations during labor to determine position of fetus.
B. Fetal shoulders: may be manipulated during delivery to allow passage of one shoulder at a time.
C. Presentation: that part of the fetus which enters the pelvis in the birth process (Figure 4-2). Types of presentation are
   1. Cephalic: head is presenting part; usually vertex (*occiput*), which is most favorable for birth. Head is flexed with chin on chest.
   2. Breech: buttocks or lower extremities present first. Types are
      a. Frank: thighs flexed, legs extended on anterior body surface, buttocks presenting
      b. Full or complete: thighs and legs flexed, buttocks and feet presenting (baby in squatting position)
      c. Footling: one or both feet are presenting

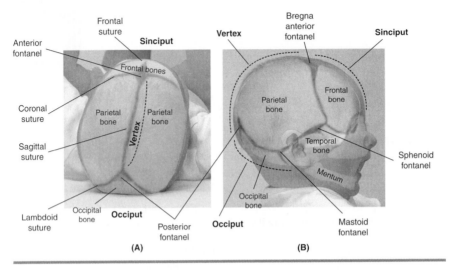

FIGURE 4-1 Fetal skull–sutures and fontanels. (A) Superior view; (B) Lateral view

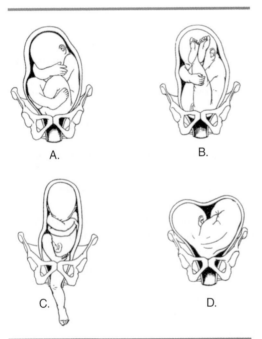

FIGURE 4-2 Breech presentations. (A) Complete; (B) Frank; (C) Footling; (D) Shoulder

3. Shoulder: presenting part is the scapula, and baby is in horizontal or transverse position. Cesarean birth indicated.

D. Position: relationship of reference point on fetal presenting part to maternal bony pelvis (Figure 4-3).

1. Maternal bony pelvis divided into four quadrants (right and left anterior; right and left posterior). Relationship is expressed in a three-letter abbreviation: first the maternal side (R or L), next the fetal presentation, and last the maternal quadrant (A or P). Most common positions are

a. LOA (left occiput anterior): fetal occiput is on maternal left side and toward front, face is down. This is a favorable delivery position.

b. ROA (right occiput anterior): fetal occiput on maternal right side toward front, face is down. This is a favorable delivery position.

c. LOP (left occiput posterior): fetal occiput is on maternal left side and toward back, face is up. Mother experiences much back discomfort during labor; labor may be slowed; rotation usually occurs before labor to anterior position, or health care provider may rotate at time of delivery.

d. ROP (right occiput posterior): fetal occiput is on maternal right side and toward back, face is up. Presents problems similar to LOP.

2. Assessment of fetal position can be made by

a. *Leopold's maneuvers*: external palpation (4 steps) of maternal abdomen to determine fetal contours or outlines. Maternal obesity, excess amniotic fluid, or uterine tumors may make palpation less accurate.

b. Vaginal examination: location of sutures and fontanels and determination of relationship to maternal bony pelvis.

c. Rectal examination: now virtually completely replaced by vaginal examination.

d. Auscultation of fetal heart tones and determination of quadrant of maternal abdomen where best heard. (Correlate with Leopold maneuvers.)

Passageway

Shape and measurement of maternal pelvis and distensibility of birth canal (see also Overview of Anatomy and Physiology.

A. Engagement: fetal presenting part enters true pelvis (inlet). May occur 2 weeks before labor in primipara; usually occurs at beginning of labor for multipara.

B. Station: measurement of how far the presenting part has descended into the pelvis. Referrant is ischial spines, palpated through lateral vaginal walls.

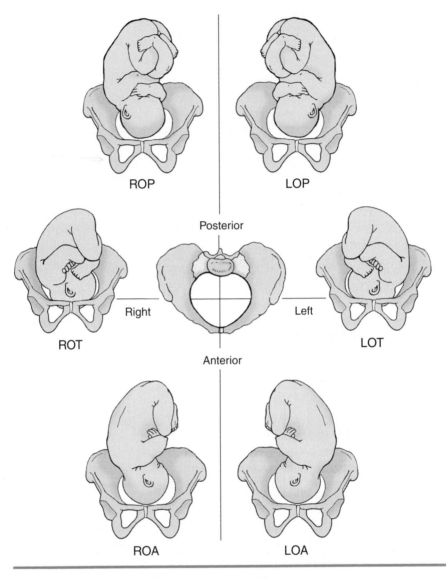

ROP LOP

Posterior

Right Left

ROT LOT

Anterior

ROA LOA

FIGURE 4-3 Positions of a vertex presentation

1. When presenting part is at ischial spines, station is 0, "engaged."
2. If presenting part is above ischial spines, station expressed as a negative number (e.g., -1, -2).
3. If presenting part is below ischial spines, station expressed as a positive number (e.g., $+1$, $+2$).
4. "High" or "floating" terms used to denote unengaged presenting part.

C. Soft tissue (cervix, vagina): stretches and dilates under the force of contractions to accommodate the passage of the fetus.

Powers

Forces of labor, acting in concert, to expel fetus and placenta. Major forces are
A. Uterine contractions (involuntary)
   1. Frequency: timed from the beginning of one contraction to the beginning of the next
   2. Regularity: discernible pattern; better established as pregnancy progresses
   3. Intensity: strength of contraction; a relative assessment without the use of a monitor. May be determined by the "depressability" of the uterus during a contraction. Described as mild, moderate, or strong.
   4. Duration: length of contraction. Contractions lasting more than 90 seconds without a subsequent period of uterine relaxation may have severe implications for the fetus and should be reported.
B. Voluntary bearing-down efforts
   1. After full dilation of the cervix, the mother can use her abdominal muscles to help expel the fetus.
   2. These efforts are similar to those for defecation, but the mother is pushing out the fetus from the birth canal.
   3. Contraction of levator ani muscles.

Placenta

A. As the placenta usually forms in the fundus of the uterus, it seldom interferes with the progress of labor.
B. A low-lying, marginal, partial, or complete placenta previa may require medical intervention to complete the birth process (see also Placenta Previa and Abruptio Placentae.

Psychologic Response

A woman who is relaxed, aware, and participating in the birth process usually has a shorter, less intense labor. A woman who is fearful has high levels of adrenaline, which slows uterine contractions.

The Labor Process

Causes

Actual cause unknown. Factors involved include
A. Progressive uterine distension
B. Increasing intrauterine pressure
C. Aging of the placenta
D. Changes in levels of estrogen, progesterone, and prostaglandins
E. Increasing myometrial irritability

Mechanisms (Vertex Presentation)

A. Engagement
   1. The biparietal diameter of the head passes the pelvic inlet.
   2. The head is fixed in the pelvis.
B. Descent: progress of the presenting part through the pelvis
C. Flexion: chin flexed more firmly onto chest by pressure on fetal head from maternal soft tissues (cervix, vaginal walls, pelvic floor)
D. Internal rotation
   1. Fetal skull rotates along axis from transverse to anteroposterior at pelvic outlet.
   2. Head passes the midpelvis.
E. Extension: head passes under the symphysis pubis and is delivered, occiput first, followed by face and chin.
F. External rotation: head rotates to full alignment with back and shoulders for shoulder delivery mechanisms.
G. *When entire body of baby has emerged from mother's body, birth is complete. This time is recorded as the time of birth.*

Stages of Labor

A. Definitions
   1. Stage 1: from onset of labor until full dilation of cervix
      a. Latent phase: from 0-4 cm
      b. Active phase: 4-8 cm
      c. Transition: 8-10 cm
   2. Stage 2: from full dilation of cervix to birth of baby
   3. Stage 3: from birth of baby to expulsion of placenta
   4. Stage 4: time after birth (usually 1-2 hours) of immediately recovery
B. Cervical changes in first stage of labor
   1. Effacement
      a. Shortening and thinning of cervix.
      b. In primipara, effacement is usually well advanced before dilation begins; in a multipara, effacement and dilation progress together.
   2. Dilation
      a. Enlargement or widening of the cervical os and canal.
      b. Full dilation is considered 10 cm.

Duration of Labor

A. Depends on
   1. Regular, progressive uterine contractions
   2. Progressive effacement and dilation of cervix
   3. Progressive descent of presenting part
B. Average length
   1. Primipara
      a. Stage 1: 12-13 hours

   b. Stage 2: 1 hour
   c. Stage 3: 3-4 minutes
   d. Stage 4: 1-2 hours
2. Multipara
   a. Stage 1: 8 hours
   b. Stage 2: 20 minutes
   c. Stage 3: 4-5 minutes
   d. Stage 4: 1-2 hours

■ ASSESSMENT DURING LABOR

Fetal Assessment

Auscultation

Auscultate FHR at least every 15-30 minutes during first stage and every 5-15 minutes during second stage (depends on risk status of client).
A. Normal range 120-160 beats/minute
B. Best recorded during the 30 seconds immediately following a contraction

Palpation

Assess intensity of contraction by manual palpation of uterine fundus.
A. Mild: tense fundus, but can be indented with fingertips.
B. Moderate: firm fundus, difficult to indent with fingertips.
C. Strong: very firm fundus, cannot indent with fingertips.

Electronic Fetal Monitoring

A. Placement of ultrasound transducer and tocotransducer to record fetal heartbeat and uterine contractions and display them on special graph paper for comparison and identification of normal and abnormal patterns.
B. Can be applied externally to mother's abdomen, or internally, within uterus.
   1. External application
      a. Less precise information collected
      b. May be affected by maternal movements
      c. Noninvasive: rupture of membranes not required, can be widely used
      d. Little danger associated with use
   2. Internal application
      a. More precise information collected
      b. Cervix must be dilated and membranes ruptured to be utilized
      c. Physician applies scalp electrode and uterine catheter
      d. Sterile technique must be maintained during application to reduce risk of intrauterine infection
      e. Can yield specific short-term variability.

C. Pattern recognition
1. Nurse is responsible for assessing FHR patterns, implementing appropriate nursing interventions, and reporting suspicious patterns to physician.
2. Baseline FHR: 120–160, when uterus is not contracting.
3. Variability is normal, indicative of intact fetal nervous system. Variability is result of interaction of sympathetic and parasympathetic nervous systems. Two types of variability are
   a. Short-term (beat-to-beat): assessed as present/absent.
   b. Long-term (rhythmic fluctuations): classified according to number of cycles/minute. Average is 6/minute.
4. Tachycardia
   a. FHR more than 160 beats/minute, lasting longer than 10 minutes.
   b. May have multiple causes.
   c. Oxygen may be administered.
5. Bradycardia
   a. FHR less than 120 beats/minute lasting longer than 10 minutes.
   b. May have multiple causes.
   c. Oxygen may be administered.
6. Early deceleration
   a. Deceleration of FHR begins early in contraction, stays within normal range, returns to baseline by end of contraction.
   b. Believed to be the result of compression of fetal head against cervix.
   c. Not an ominous pattern, no nursing interventions required.
7. Late deceleration
   a. Deceleration of FHR begins late in contraction; depth varies with strength of contraction; does not return to baseline by end of contraction.
   b. May be occasional or consistent. Gradual increase in number is always suspicious and MUST be reported/charted.
   c. Believed to be the result of uteroplacental insufficiency.
   d. **An ominous pattern**.
   e. Nurse should place in side-lying position, administer oxygen, discontinue any oxytocin infusion, assess variability, prepare for immediate delivery if pattern remains uncorrected.
8. Variable deceleration
   a. Onset of deceleration not related to uterine contraction.
   b. Swings in FHR abrupt and dramatic, return to baseline frequently rapid.
   c. Believed to be the result of compression of the umbilical cord.
   d. **Although not an ominous pattern, continued nursing assessment required**.
   e. Nurse should change maternal position to relieve pressure on cord; if no improvement seen, administer oxygen, discontinue

oxytocin if infusing, prepare client for vaginal exam to assess for prolapsed cord (see also Prolapsed Umbilical Cord.

    f. If cord is prolapsed, relieve pressure on cord; do not attempt to replace cord.

    g. Cesarean delivery will be needed.

Maternal Assessment

Premonitory Assessment

Physiologic changes preceding labor

A. Lightening (engagement): occurs up to two weeks before labor in primipara; at beginning of labor for multipara

B. Braxton Hicks' contractions: may become more noticeable; may play a part in ripening of cervix

C. Easier respirations from decreased pressure on diaphragm

D. Frequent urination, from increased pressure on bladder

E. Restlessness/poor sleeping patterns, "nesting" behaviors

True vs False Labor

A. True labor
1. Contractions increased in frequency, intensity, and duration
2. Progressive cervical changes
3. Bloody show
4. Progressive fetal descent
5. Walking intensifies contractions
6. Discomfort begins in back then radiates to abdomen

B. False labor
1. Irregular, inefficient contractions not causing the progressive changes associated with true labor
2. No bloody show
3. Discomfort primarily in abdomen, may be relieved by walking
4. Need to assess client over period of time to differentiate from true labor

■ FIRST STAGE OF LABOR

Latent Phase (0–4 cm)

Assessment

A. Contractions: frequency, intensity, duration

B. Membranes: intact or ruptured, color of fluid

C. Bloody show

D. Time of onset

E. Cervical changes

F. Time of last ingestion of food

G. FHR every 15 minutes; immediately after rupture of membranes

H. Maternal vital signs
   1. Temperature every 2 hours if membranes ruptured, every 4 hours if intact
   2. Pulse and respirations every hour or prn as indicated
   3. Blood pressure every half hour or prn as indicated
I. Progress of descent (station)
J. Client's knowledge of labor process
K. Client's affect
L. Client's birth plan

Analysis

Nursing diagnoses for the latent phase of first stage of labor may include
A. Anxiety
B. Ineffective breathing pattern
C. Pain
D. Deficient knowledge

Planning and Implementation

A. Goals
   1. Complete all admission procedures.
   2. Labor will progress normally.
   3. Mother/fetus will tolerate latent phase successfully.
B. Interventions
   1. Administer perineal prep/enema if ordered/appropriate.
   2. Assess vital signs, blood pressure, fetal heart, contractions, bloody show, cervical changes, descent of fetus as scheduled.
   3. Maintain bed rest if indicated or required.
   4. Reinforce/teach breathing techniques as needed.
   5. Support laboring woman/couple based on their needs.
   6. Have client attempt to void every 1-2 hours.
   7. Apply external fetal monitoring if indicated or ordered.

Evaluation

A. Admission procedures complete
B. Progress through latent stage normal, cervix dilated
C. Mother/fetus tolerate latent phase well, mother as comfortable as possible, vital signs normal; FHR maintained in response to contractions

Active Phase (4–8 cm)

Assessment

A. Cervical changes
B. Bloody show
C. Membranes

D. Progress of descent
E. Maternal/fetal vital signs
F. Client's affect

Analysis

Nursing diagnoses for the active phase of first stage of labor may include
A. Ineffective coping
B. Impaired oral mucous membranes
C. Deficient knowledge
D. Pain
E. Ineffective tissue perfusion
F. Risk for injury

Planning and Implementation

A. Goals
  1. Progress will be normal through active phase.
  2. Mother/fetus will successfully complete active phase.
B. Interventions
  1. Continue to observe labor progress.
  2. Reinforce/teach breathing techniques as needed.
  3. Position client for maximum comfort.
  4. Support client/couple as mother becomes more involved in labor.
  5. Administer analgesia if ordered or indicated.
  6. Assist with anesthesia if given and monitor maternal/fetal vital signs.
  7. Provide ice chips or clear fluids for mother to drink if allowed/desired.
  8. Keep client/couple informed as labor progresses.
  9. With posterior position, apply sacral counterpressure, or have father do so.

Evaluation

A. Labor progressing through active phase, dilation progressing
B. Mother/fetus tolerating labor appropriately
C. No complications observed

Transition (8–10 cm)

Assessment

A. Progress of labor
B. Cervical changes
C. Maternal mood changes: if irritable or aggressive may be tiring or unable to cope
D. Signs of nausea, vomiting, trembling, crying, irritability
E. Maternal/fetal vital signs
F. Breathing patterns, may be hyperventilating
G. Urge to bear down with contractions

Analysis

Nursing diagnoses for the transition phase of first stage of labor may include
A. Ineffective breathing pattern
B. Powerlessness
C. Ineffective coping

Planning and Implementation

A. Goals
  1. Labor will continue to progress through transition.
  2. Mother/fetus will tolerate process well.
  3. Complications will be avoided.
B. Interventions
  1. Continue observation of labor progress, maternal/fetal vital signs.
  2. Give mother positive support if tired or discouraged.
  3. Accept behavioral changes of mother.
  4. Promote appropriate breathing patterns to prevent hyperventilation.
  5. If hyperventilation present, have mother rebreathe expelled carbon dioxide to reverse respiratory alkalosis.
  6. Discourage pushing efforts until cervix is completely dilated, then assist with pushing.
  7. Observe for signs of delivery.

Evaluation

A. Mother/fetus progressed through transition
B. No complications observed
C. Mother/fetus ready for second stage of labor

■ SECOND STAGE OF LABOR

Assessment

A. Signs of imminent delivery
B. Progress of descent
C. Maternal/fetal vital signs
D. Maternal pushing efforts
E. Vaginal distension
F. Bulging of perineum
G. Crowning
H. Birth of baby

Analysis

Nursing diagnoses for the second stage of labor may include
A. Risk for injury
B. Noncompliance related to exhaustion
C. Deficient knowledge

Planning and Implementation

A. Goals
  1. Safe delivery of living, uninjured fetus.
  2. Mother will be comfortable after tolerating delivery.

B. Interventions
  1. If necessary, transfer mother carefully to delivery table or birthing chair; support legs equally to prevent/minimize strain on ligaments.
  2. Carefully position mother on delivery table, in delivery chair, or birthing bed to prevent popliteal vein pressure.
  3. Help mother use handles or legs to pull on as she bears down with contractions.
  4. Clean vulva and perineum to prepare for delivery.
  5. Continue observation of maternal/fetal vital signs.
  6. Encourage mother in sustained (5–7 seconds) pushes with each contraction.
  7. Support father's participation if in delivery area.
  8. Catheterize mother's bladder if indicated.
  9. Keep mother informed of delivery progress.
  10. Note time of delivery of baby.

Evaluation

A. Delivery of healthy viable fetus
B. Mother comfortable after procedure
C. No complications during procedure

■ THIRD STAGE OF LABOR

Assessment

A. Signs of placental separation
  1. Gush of blood
  2. Lengthening of cord
  3. Change in shape of uterus (discoid to globular)
B. Completeness of placenta
C. Status of mother/baby contact for first critical 1–2 hours
  1. Baby's Apgar scores (see Table 4-1)
  2. Blood pressure, pulse, respirations, lochia, fundal status of mother

Analysis

Nursing diagnoses for the third stage of labor may include
A. Pain
B. Risk for deficient fluid volume

TABLE 4-1   Apgar Scoring

Category	0	1	2	Score
Heart rate	Absent	<100	>100	——
Respiratory effort	Absent	Slow, irregular	Good cry	——
Muscle tone	Absent/ limp	Some flexion	Active motion	——
Reflex irritability	No response	Grimace	Cry	——
Color	Blue, pale	Body pink, extremities blue	All pink	——
			Total Score	——

Planning and Implementation

A. Goals
  1. Placenta will be delivered without complications.
  2. Maternal blood loss will be minimized.
  3. Mother will tolerate procedures well.
B. Interventions
  1. Palpate fundus immediately after delivery of placenta; massage gently if not firm.
  2. Palpate fundus at least every 15 minutes for first 1-2 hours.
  3. Observe lochia for color and amount.
  4. Inspect perineum.
  5. Assist with maternal hygiene as needed.
     a. Clean gown.
     b. Warm blanket.
     c. Clean perineal pads.
  6. Offer fluids as indicated.
  7. Promote beginning relationship with baby and parents through touch and privacy.
  8. Administer medications as ordered/needed (pitocin added to IV if present).

Evaluation

A. Placenta delivered without complications
B. Minimal maternal blood loss
C. Mother tolerated procedure well

■ FOURTH STAGE OF LABOR

Assessment

A. Fundal firmness, position
B. Lochia: color, amount
C. Perineum
D. Vital signs
E. IV if running
F. Infant's heart rate, airway, color, muscle tone, reflexes, warmth, activity state
G. Bonding/family integration

Analysis

Nursing diagnoses for the fourth stage of labor may include
A. Pain
B. Risk for deficient fluid volume
C. Interrupted family processes

Planning and Implementation

A. Goal: critical first hour(s) after delivery will pass without complications for mother/baby.
B. Interventions
   1. Palpate fundus every 15 minutes for first 1-2 hours; massage gently if not firm.
   2. Check mother's blood pressure, pulse, respirations every 15 minutes for first 1-2 hours or until stable.
   3. Check lochia for color and amount every 15 minutes for first 1-2 hours.
   4. Inspect perineum every 15 minutes for first 1-2 hours.
   5. Apply ice to perineum if swollen or if episiotomy.
   6. Encourage mother to void, particularly if fundus not firm or displaced.
      a. Use nursing techniques to encourage voiding.
      b. If client unable to void, get order for catheterization.
      c. Measure first voiding.
   7. Encourage early bonding; through breastfeeding if desired.

Evaluation

A. Mother's vital signs stable, fundus and lochia within normal limits
B. Evidence of bonding; parents cuddle, touch, talk to baby
C. No complications observed for mother or baby during crucial time

■ COMPLICATIONS OF LABOR AND DELIVERY
Premature/Preterm Labor

A. General information
   1. Labor that occurs before the end of the 37th week of pregnancy.
   2. Cause is frequently unknown, but the following conditions are associated with premature labor
      a. Cervical incompetence
      b. Preeclampsia/eclampsia
      c. Maternal injury
      d. Infection (urinary tract infection)
      e. Multiple gestation, polyhydramnios
      f. Placental disorders
   3. Preterm labor: prevention
      a. Minimize or stop smoking: a major factor in preterm labor and birth.
      b. Minimize or stop substance abuse/chemical dependency.
      c. Early and consistent prenatal care.
      d. Appropriate diet/weight gain.
      e. Minimize psychological stressors.
      f. Minimize/prevent exposure to infections.
      g. Learn to recognize signs and symptoms of preterm labor.
   4. Incidence of preterm labor is between 5% and 10% in all pregnancies and is a major cause of perinatal mortality.
B. Medical management
   1. Unless labor is irreversible, or a condition exists in which the mother or fetus would be jeopardized by the continuation of the pregnancy, or the membranes have ruptured, the usual medical intervention is to attempt to arrest the premature labor (tocolysis).
   2. Medications used in the treatment of premature labor
      a. Magnesium sulfate
         1) stops uterine contractions with fewer side effects than beta-adrenergic drugs.
         2) interferes with muscle contractility.
         3) administered IV for 12 to 24 hours, PO form of magnesium may be used for maintenance.
            a) loading dose of 4-6 grams IV over 20 to 30 minutes
            b) maintenance dose IV 1-3 g/hr (IV piggyback)
            c) must monitor client for magnesium toxicity
         4) few serious side effects; initially client feels hot, flushed, sweats, may c/o headache, nausea, diarrhea, dizziness, nystagmus, and lethargy.
         5) most serious side effect: respiratory depression.
         6) most common fetal side effect is hypotonia.

      b. Beta-adrenergic drugs—Terbutaline and Ritodrine.
- **1)** decreases effect of calcium on muscle activation to slow or stop uterine contractions.
- **2)** initially given IV, then PO brethine (terbutaline) for maintenance.
- **3)** terbutaline:
  - **a)** 1-8 mg/min $\times$ 8-12 hr
  - **b)** 2.5 to 5 mg PO q 4-8 hr
- **4)** ritodrine
  - **a)** 0.05-0.1 mg/min increased to 0.35 mg/min until contractions stop.
  - **b)** 10-20 mg q 2 h for 24 hours
- **5)** side effects: increased heart rate, nervousness, tremors, nausea and vomiting, decrease in serum K+ level, cardiac arrhythmias, pulmonary edema.

      c. Nifedipine
- **1)** calcium channel blocker
- **2)** 10-30 mg loading dose, oral or sublingual; second dose may be given in 30 min if contractions persist; 10-20 mg orally q 4-6 hr for maintenance.
- **3)** side effects: facial flushing, mild hypotension, reflex tachycardia, headache, nausea.

      d. Indomethacin
- **1)** prostaglandin synthetase inhibitor
- **2)** loading dose: 50-100 mg PO or rectally: 25 mg q 4-6 hr for 24-48 hr maintenance
- **3)** side effects: nausea, vomiting, dyspepsia

3. When premature labor cannot or should not be arrested and fetal lung maturity needs to be improved, the use of betamethasone (Celestone) can improve the L/S ratio of lung surfactants. It is administered IM to the mother, usually every 12 hr times 2, then weekly until 34 weeks' gestation.

C. Nursing interventions
1. Keep client at rest, side-lying position.
2. Hydrate the client and maintain with IV or PO fluids.
3. Maintain continuous maternal/fetal monitoring.

      a. Maternal/fetal vital signs every 10 minutes; be alert for abrupt changes.
      b. Monitor maternal I&O.
      c. Monitor urine for glucose and ketones.
      d. Watch cardiac and respiratory status carefully.
      e. Evaluate lab test results carefully.

4. Administer drugs as ordered/indicated.
      a. Terbutaline
- **1)** position client on side as much as possible.

CLIENT TEACHING CHECKLIST

If the client is at home, advise her to:

- Maintain bed rest until symptoms subside. Resume activities slowly once symptoms have subsided
- Drink 3–4 glasses of water or juice daily
- Empty bladder
- Rest on left side
- Avoid sexual intercourse

Call health care provider immediately if:

- Symptoms have not subsided or if symptoms return
- Contractions are every 5 minutes or less
- Vaginal bleeding occurs
- Odorous vaginal discharge occurs
- Fluid is leaking from the vagina

      2) apply external fetal monitor.

      3) complete maternal/fetal assessment before each increase in dosage rate.

      4) special maternal assessment includes respiratory status, blood pressure, pulse, I&O, lab values.

      5) notify physician of significant changes.

      6) support client through stressful period of treatment and uncertainty.

      7) teach client necessity of continuing oral medication at home if discharged.

    b. Magnesium sulfate: carefully monitor respirations, reflexes, and urinary output (see also Severe Preeclampsia.

  5. Keep client informed of all progress/changes.

  6. Identify side effects/complications as early as possible.

  7. Carry out activities designed to keep client comfortable.

Postmature/Prolonged Pregnancy

A. General information

  1. Defined as those pregnancies lasting beyond the end of the 42nd week.

  2. Fetus at risk due to placental degeneration and loss of amniotic fluid (cord accidents).

  3. Decreased amounts of vernix also allow the drying of the fetal skin, resulting in a dry, parchmentlike skin condition.

B. Medical management
   1. Directed toward ascertaining precise fetal gestational age and condition, and determining fetal ability to tolerate labor
   2. Induction of labor and possibly cesarean birth
C. Assessment findings
   1. Measurements of fetal gestational age for fetal maturity
   2. Biophysical profile
D. Nursing interventions
   1. Perform continual monitoring of maternal/fetal vital signs.
   2. Support mother through all testing and labor
   3. Assist with amnio-infusion if ordered to increase cushion for cord.

Prolapsed Umbilical Cord

A. General information
   1. Displacement of cord in a downward direction, near or ahead of the presenting part, or into the vagina
   2. May occur when membranes rupture, or with ensuing contractions
   3. Associated with breech presentations, unengaged presentations, and premature labors
   4. Obstetric emergency: if compression of the cord occurs, fetal hypoxia may result in CNS damage or death.
B. Assessment findings: vaginal exam identifies cord prolapse into vagina
C. Nursing interventions
   1. Check fetal heart tones immediately when membranes rupture, and again after next contraction, or within 5 minutes; report decelerations.
   2. If fetal bradycardia, perform vaginal examination and check for prolapsed cord.
   3. If cord prolapsed into vagina, exert upward pressure against presenting part to lift part off cord, reducing pressure on cord.
   4. Get help to move mother into a position where gravity assists in getting presenting part off cord (knee-chest position or severe Trendelenburg's).
   5. Administer oxygen, and prepare for immediate cesarean birth.
   6. If cord protrudes outside vagina, cover with sterile gauze moistened with sterile saline while carrying out above tasks. Do not attempt to replace cord.
   7. Notify physician.

Premature Rupture of Membranes

A. General information
   1. Loss of amniotic fluid, prior to term, unconnected with labor.
   2. Dangers associated with this event are prolapsed cord, infection, and the potential need for premature delivery.

B. Assessment findings
   1. Report from mother/family of discharge of fluid.
   2. pH of vaginal fluid will differentiate between amniotic fluid (alkaline) and urine or purulent discharge (acidic).
C. Nursing interventions
   1. Monitor maternal/fetal vital signs on continuous basis, especially maternal temperature.
   2. Calculate gestational age.
   3. Observe for signs of infection and for signs of onset of labor.
      a. If signs of infection present, administer antibiotics as ordered and prepare for immediate delivery.
      b. If no maternal infection, induction of labor may be delayed.
   4. Observe and record color, odor, amount of amniotic fluid.
   5. Examine mother for signs of prolapsed cord.
   6. Provide explanations of procedures and findings, and support mother/family.
   7. Prepare mother/family for early birth if indicated.

Fetal Distress

A. General information: common contributing factors are
   1. Cord compression.
   2. Placental abnormalities.
   3. Preexisting maternal disease.
B. Assessment findings
   1. Decelerations in FHR
   2. Meconium-stained amniotic fluid with a vertex presentation
   3. Fetal scalp sampling (may be needed for a definitive diagnosis)
C. Nursing interventions
   1. Check FHR on appropriate basis, institute fetal monitoring if not already in use.
   2. Conduct vaginal exam for presentation and position.
   3. Place mother on left side, administer oxygen, check for prolapsed cord, notify physician.
   4. Support mother and family
   5. Prepare for emergency birth if indicated.

Dystocia

A. General information
   1. Any labor/delivery that is prolonged or difficult
   2. Usually results from a change in the interrelationships among the 5 Ps (factors in labor/delivery): *p*assenger, *p*assage, *p*owers, *p*lacenta, and *p*syche of mother.
   3. Frequently seen causes include

    a. Disproportion between fetal presentation (usually the head) and maternal pelvis (cephalopelvic disproportion [CPD]).
      1) if disproportion is minimal, vaginal birth may be attempted if fetal injuries can be minimized or eliminated.
      2) cesarean birth needed if disproportion is great.
    b. Problems with presentation
      1) any presentation unfavorable for delivery (e.g., breech, shoulder, face, transverse lie)
      2) posterior presentation that does not rotate, or cannot be rotated with ease.
      3) cesarean birth is the usual intervention.
    c. Problems with maternal soft tissue
      1) a full bladder may impede the progress of labor, as can myomata uteri, cervical edema, scar tissue, and congenital anomalies.
      2) emptying the bladder may allow labor to continue; the other conditions may necessitate cesarean birth.
    d. Dysfunctional uterine contractions
      1) contractions may be too weak, too short, too far apart, ineffectual.
      2) progress of labor is affected; progressive dilation, effacement, and descent do not occur in the expected pattern.
      3) Classification
        a) primary: inefficient pattern present from beginning of labor; usually a prolonged latent phase.
        b) secondary: efficient pattern that changes to inefficient or stops; may occur in any stage.
B. Assessment findings
    1. Progress of labor slower than expected rate of dilation, effacement, descent for specific client
    2. Length of labor prolonged
    3. Maternal exhaustion/distress
    4. Fetal distress
C. Nursing interventions
    1. Individualized as to cause.
    2. Provide comfort measures for client.
    3. Provide clear, supportive descriptions of all actions taken.
    4. Administer analgesia if ordered/indicated.
    5. Prepare oxytocin infusion for induction of labor if ordered.
    6. Monitor mother/fetus continuously.
    7. Prepare for cesarean birth if needed.

Precipitous Labor and Delivery

A. General information
    1. Labor of less than 3 hours.
    2. Emergency delivery without client's physician or midwife

TABLE 4-2   Emergency Delivery of an Infant

If you have to deliver the baby yourself
- Assess the client's affect and ability to understand directions, as well as other resources available (other physicians, nurses, auxiliary personnel).
- Stay with client at all times; mother must not be left alone if delivery is imminent.
- Do not prevent birth of baby.
- Maintain sterile environment if possible.
- Rupture membranes if necessary.
- Support baby's head as it emerges, preventing too-rapid delivery with gentle pressure.
- Check for nuchal cord, slip over head if possible.
- Use gentle aspiration with bulb syringe to remove blood and mucus from nose and mouth.
- Deliver shoulders after external rotation, asking mother to push gently if needed.
- Provide support for baby's body as it is delivered.
- Hold baby in head-down position to facilitate drainage of secretions.
- Promote cry by gently rubbing over back and soles of feet.
- Dry to prevent heat loss.
- Place baby on mother's abdomen.
- Check for signs of placental separation.
- Check mother for excess bleeding; massage uterus prn.
- Hold placenta as it is delivered.
- Cut cord when pulsations cease, if cord clamp is available; if no clamps, leave intact.
- Wrap baby in dry blanket, give to mother; put to breast if possible.
- Check mother for fundal firmness and excess bleeding.
- Record all pertinent data.
- Comfort mother and family as needed.

B. Assessment findings
  1. As labor is progressing quickly, assessment may need to be done rapidly.
  2. Client may have history of previous precipitous labor and delivery.
  3. Desire to push.
  4. Observe status of membranes, perineal area for bulging, and for signs of bleeding.
C. Nursing interventions (see Table 4-2)

Amniotic Fluid Embolism

A. General information
  1. Escape of amniotic fluid into the maternal circulation, usually in conjunction with a pattern of hypertonic, intense uterine contractions, either naturally or oxytocin induced.
  2. Obstetric emergency: may be fatal to the mother and to the baby.

B. Assessment findings
   1. Sudden onset of respiratory distress, hypotension, chest pain, signs of shock
   2. Bleeding (DIC)
   3. Cyanosis
   4. Pulmonary edema
C. Nursing interventions
   1. Initiate emergency life support activities for mother.
      a. Administer oxygen
      b. Utilize CPR in case of cardiac arrest.
   2. Establish IV line for blood transfusion and monitoring of CVP.
   3. Administer medications to control bleeding as ordered.
   4. Prepare for emergency birth of baby.
   5. Keep client/family informed as possible.

Induction of Labor

A. General information: deliberate stimulation of uterine contractions before the normal occurrence of labor.
B. Medical management: may be accomplished by
   1. Amniotomy (the deliberate rupture of membranes)
   2. Oxytocins, usually Pitocin
   3. Prostaglandin (PGE_2) in gel/suppository form to improve cervical readiness
C. Assessment findings
   1. Indications for use
      a. Postmature pregnancy
      b. Preeclampsia/eclampsia
      c. Diabetes
      d. Premature rupture of membranes
   2. Condition of fetus: mature, engaged vertex fetus in no distress
   3. Condition of mother: cervix "ripe" for induction, no CPD
D. Nursing interventions
   1. Explain all procedures to client.
   2. Prepare appropriate equipment and medications.
      a. Amniotomy: a small tear made in amniotic membrane as part of sterile vaginal exam
         1) explain sensations to client.
         2) check FHR immediately before and after procedure; marked changes may indicate prolapsed cord (see page 571).
         3) additional care as for woman with premature rupture of membranes.
      b. Oxytocin (Pitocin): IV administration, "piggybacked" to main IV

1) usual dilution 10 mU/1000 ml fluid, delivered via infusion pump for greatest accuracy in controlling dosage.
2) usual administration rate is 0.5-1.0 mU/min, increased no more than 1-2 mU/min at 40-60-minute intervals until regular pattern of appropriate contractions is established (every 2-3 minutes, lasting less than 90 seconds, with 30-45 second rest period between contractions).

3. Know that continuous monitoring and accurate assessments are essential.
   a. Apply external continuous fetal monitoring equipment.
   b. Monitor maternal condition on a continuous basis: blood pressure, pulse, progress of labor.
4. Discontinue oxytocin infusion when
   a. Fetal distress is noted.
   b. Hypertonic contractions occur.
   c. Signs of other obstetric complications (hemorrhage/shock, abruptio placenta, amniotic fluid embolism) appear.
5. Notify physician of any untoward reactions.

■ ANALGESIA AND ANESTHESIA

Analgesia for Labor

General Information

A. Definition: the easing of pain or discomfort by the administration of medication that blocks pain recognition or the raising of the pain recognition threshold.
B. Sources of pain/discomfort
   1. First stage of labor: stretching of cervix and uterine contractions
   2. Second stage of labor: stretching of birth canal and perineum
C. Examples of medications used systemically for labor analgesia
   1. Sedatives: help to relieve anxiety; may use secobarbital (Seconal), sodium pentobarbital (Nembutal), phenobarbital.
   2. Narcotic analgesics: help to relieve pain; may use morphine, meperidine (Demerol), butorphanol (Stadol), fentanyl (Sublimaze), nalbuphine hydrochloride (Nubain).
   3. Narcotic antagonists: given to reverse narcotic depression of mother or baby; may use naloxone (Narcan), levallorphan (Lorfan).
   4. Analgesic potentiating drugs: given to raise desired effect of analgesic without raising dose of analgesic drug; may use promethazine (Phenergan), promazine (Sparine), propiomazine (Largon), hydroxyzine (Vistaril)
D. Medication administration
   1. IV: the preferred route; allows for smaller doses, better control of administration, better prediction of action.

NURSING ALERT

A nalgesic agents may decrease contraction frequency and intensity; this may result in neonatal respiratory depression.

DELEGATION TIP

V ital signs assessment may be delegated to assistive personnel. Ancillary personnel are generally informed about the medications the client is receiving and if adverse effects are anticipated or being monitored.

2. IM: still widely used; needs larger dose, absorption may be delayed or erratic.
3. SC: used occasionally for small doses of nonirritating drugs.

Assessment
A. Client's perception of pain/discomfort
B. Baseline vital signs for later comparison
C. Known allergies
D. Current status of labor: medications best given in active phase of first stage of labor
E. Time of previous doses of medications

Analysis
Nursing diagnoses for labor analgesia may include
A. Pain
B. Ineffective coping
C. Deficient knowledge

Planning and Implementation
A. Goals
  1. Medication will relieve maternal discomfort.
  2. Maternal comfort will be achieved with least effect of medication on fetus.
B. Interventions
  1. Administer medications on schedule to maximize maternal effect and minimize fetal effect.
  2. Continue to observe maternal/fetal vital signs for side effects.
  3. Explain to client that she must remain in bed with side rails up.
  4. Record accurately drug used, time, amount, route, site, and client response.

Evaluation
A. Medication exerts intended effect.
B. Mother reports positive response to medication.
C. Fetus shows no ill effects from medication.
D. Labor is not affected by medication.

Anesthesia for Labor and Delivery

General Information
A. Removal of pain perception by the administration of medication to interrupt the transmission of nerve impulses to the brain.
B. May be administered by inhalation, IV, or regional routes.
C. All methods of labor and delivery anesthesia have their drawbacks; no one method is perfect.
D. Types of labor and delivery anesthesia
  1. Inhalation: mother inhales controlled concentration of gaseous medication.
    a. Administered by trained personnel only
    b. Methoxyflurane (Penthrane) and nitrous oxide commonly used
    c. Dangers include regurgitation and aspiration, uterine relaxation, and hemorrhage postdelivery.
  2. IV: rarely used in uncomplicated vaginal deliveries; may be used for cesarean birth (as induction anesthesia).
    a. Administered by trained personnel only
    b. Sodium pentothal commonly used
  3. Regional: medication introduced to specific areas to block pain impulses
    a. Always administered by skilled personnel
    b. Medications used include tetracaine (Pontocaine), lidocaine, bupivacaine (Marcaine), mepivacaine (Carbocaine)
    c. May block nerve at the root or in a peripheral area
      1) nerve root blocks
        a) *lumbar epidural*: may be given continuously or intermittently during labor, or at time of delivery; medication is injected over dura through lumbar interspace; absorption of drug is slower, with less hypotension; client should have no postspinal headache
        b) *caudal*: may be given intermittently through labor, or at time of delivery; medication is injected through sacral hiatus into peridural space; client should have no postspinal headache
        c) *subarachnoid (low spinal, saddle block)*: given when delivery is imminent; medication is injected into spinal fluid; mother may experience postdelivery headache;

keep flat for at least 6–8 hours postspinal and encourage oral fluids postdelivery to facilitate reversal of headache.
   2) peripheral nerve blocks
      a) *paracervical*: instillation of medication into cervix; rarely used during labor because of effect on fetus; useful only in first stage of labor.
      b) *pudendal*: medication injected transvaginally to affect pudendal nerve as it passes behind ischial spines on either side of vagina; useful for delivery and episiotomy if needed.
      c) *perineal (local)*: injected into the perineum at the time of delivery in order to perform an episiotomy

Assessment

A. Status of labor progress
B. Maternal/fetal vital signs
C. Allergies
D. Effects of medication on client (she may need help pushing)
E. Level of anesthesia
F. Return of sensation after anesthesia

Analysis

Nursing diagnoses for anesthesia during labor and delivery may include
A. Impaired mobility
B. Ineffective tissue perfusion
C. Deficient knowledge
D. Impaired urinary elimination

Planning and Implementation

A. Goals
   1. Pain relief will be obtained.
   2. Healthy maternal/fetal status will be maintained.
B. Interventions
   1. Assist client to empty bladder.
   2. Assist client to assume appropriate position.
      a. Inhalation anesthesia: supine with wedge under right hip to displace gravid uterus off inferior vena cava
      b. Pudendal and perineal: on back or left side
      c. Other regional types: on left side or sitting up
   3. Check maternal blood pressure and fetal heart rate every 3–5 minutes until stable, then every 15 minutes or prn.
   4. If blood pressure drops, turn client on left side, administer oxygen, and notify physician.

NURSING ALERT

P ost lumbar epidural, monitor urinary output to prevent urinary retention and monitor blood pressure to prevent hypotension.

Evaluation
A. Client experiences expected pain relief.
B. Fetus exhibits no untoward effects, FHTs remain relatively stable.
C. Labor and delivery carried out as expected.
D. Client's vital signs remain within normal limits.

■ OPERATIVE OBSTETRICAL PROCEDURES

Episiotomy
A. General information
   1. Incision made in the perineum to enlarge the vaginal opening for delivery
   2. Client usually anesthetized in some manner
   3. Types
      a. Midline or median: from posterior vaginal opening through center of perineum toward anal sphincter.
         1) most frequently used
         2) easily done, least discomfort for client
         3) danger of extension into anal sphincter
      b. Mediolateral: begins at posterior vaginal opening but angles off to left or right at $45°$ angle (rarely in the United States).
         1) done when need for additional enlargement of vaginal opening is a possibility
         2) mediolateral episiotomy usually more uncomfortable than median
   4. Advantages of episiotomy are
      a. Enlarging of vaginal opening
      b. Second stage of labor shortened
      c. Stretching of perineal muscles minimized
      d. Tearing of perineum may be prevented
   5. Those opposed to episiotomies argue
      a. Kegel exercises can prepare the perineum to stretch for delivery.
      b. Lacerations may occur anyway.
   6. Side-lying delivery minimizes the strain on the perineum and may, if used, reduce incidence of episiotomies.
B. Nursing interventions
   1. Apply ice packs to perineal area in first 12 hours to help alleviate pain and swelling.
   2. Help promote healing with warm sitz baths after first 12 hours.

3. Observe episiotomy site for signs of infection or hematoma.
4. Instruct client about perineal hygiene.

Assisted Delivery: Vacuum or Forceps

A. General information
   1. Used when there is a need to shorten the second stage or the second stage has stopped. Reasons include maternal fatigue, medical conditions, fetal distress, poor pushing, and excessive infant size.
   2. Prerequisites include: head is engaged, no CPD, membranes ruptured, cervix completely dilated, empty bladder.
B. Types of assisted deliveries
   1. Low outlet forceps used when the head is visible at the perineum.
   2. Mid and high forceps no longer used.
   3. Vacuum extraction used when head is visible—silastic suction cup applied to presenting part and gentle traction exerted while mother pushes.
C. Nursing interventions
   1. Anticipate request for forceps if possible.
   2. Monitor FHTs continuously.
   3. Explain procedure to client if awake, advise mother/family about possible presence of bruising that will go away but may contribute to jaundice, also risk of perineal or vaginal tearing.
   4. Newborn assessment should include careful examination for bruising and facial nerve damage with forceps and cephalhematoma with vacuum.
   5. Ongoing newborn assessment includes careful checking for jaundice.

Cesarean Birth

General Information

A. Delivery of the baby through an incision into the abdominal and uterine walls
B. Indications
   1. Fetal distress, disease, or anomaly
   2. Breech or other malpresentation, cephalopelvic disproportion, macrosomia
   3. Placenta previa or abruptio
   4. Prolapsed cord and other obstetric emergencies
   5. Failure to progress in labor
   6. Multiple gestation
   7. Maternal disease
   8. Previous uterine surgery
   9. Active herpes

C. Types
   1. Classical: vertical incisions made into both abdomen and uterus
      a. Used when rapid delivery is important, as in fetal distress, prolapsed cord, placenta abruptio
      b. Maternal bleeding greater with this method; client may have increased risk of uterine rupture of scar tissue with future pregnancies; not usually a candidate for vaginal birth in future pregnancies.
   2. Low cervical/low segment: transverse incisions made in abdomen (above pubic hairline) and in uterus
      a. Most common method used
      b. Procedure may take longer than classic because of need to deflect bladder, but blood loss is lessened and adhesions are fewer.
      c. Vaginal birth after this type of cesarean birth (VBAC) is a possibility.

Preoperative

A. Assessment
   1. Maternal/fetal responses to labor
   2. Indications for cesarean birth
   3. Blood and urine test results
B. Analysis: nursing diagnoses for the preoperative phase of cesarean birth may include
   1. Fear
   2. Knowledge deficit
   3. Powerlessness
   4. Disturbance in self-concept
C. Planning and implementation
   1. Goals
      a. Client prepared for surgery carefully and competently.
      b. Client will have procedures explained to her.
   2. Interventions
      a. Shave/prep abdomen and pubic area.
      b. Insert retention catheter into bladder.
      c. Administer preoperative medications as ordered.
      d. Explain all procedures to client.
      e. Provide emotional support to client/family as needed.
      f. Complete all preoperative charting responsibilities.
D. Evaluation
   1. Client adequately prepared for surgery
   2. Client understands all procedures

Postoperative

A. Assessment
   1. Maternal vital signs

2. Observation of incision for signs of infection
3. I&O
4. Level of consciousness/return of sensation
5. Fundal firmness and location
6. Lochia: color, amount, clots, odor

B. Analysis: nursing diagnoses postoperatively for cesarean birth may include
1. Alteration in comfort: pain
2. High risk for fluid volume deficit
3. High risk for alteration in parenting
4. Altered family processes

C. Planning and implementation
1. Goals
a. Healing will be promoted.
b. Bonding between mother/couple and baby will be promoted.
c. No complications will ensue.
2. Interventions
a. Implement general postsurgical care, and general postpartum care.
b. Assist client with self-care as needed.
c. Assist mother with baby care and handling as needed.
d. Encourage client to verbalize reaction to all events.
e. Reinforce any special discharge instructions from physician.

D. Evaluation
1. Mother and baby tolerated procedures well
2. No postoperative complications or infection
3. Maternal/newborn bonding occurring

REVIEW QUESTIONS

1. The nurse is caring for a woman who is admitted to the hospital in active labor. What information is most important for the nurse to assess to avoid respiratory complications during labor and delivery?

   1. Family history of lung disease.
   2. Food or drug allergies.
   3. Number of cigarettes smoked daily.
   4. When the client last ate.

2. A woman who is gravida 1 is in the active phase of stage 1 labor. The fetal position is LOA. When her membranes rupture, the nurse should expect to see

   1. a large amount of bloody fluid.
   2. a moderate amount of clear to straw-colored fluid.

   3. a small amount of greenish fluid.

   4. a small segment of the umbilical cord.

3. The nurse is caring for a woman in stage 1 labor. The fetal position is LOA. When her membranes rupture, the nurse's first action should be to

   1. notify the physician.

   2. measure the amount of fluid.

   3. count the fetal heart rate.

   4. perform a vaginal examination.

4. A woman has just delivered a 9 lb 10 oz baby. After the delivery, the nurse notices that the mother is chilly and that her fundus has relaxed. The nurse administers the oxytocin that the physician orders. The nurse knows that it has had the expected effect when

   1. the mother states that she feels warmer now.

   2. the mother falls asleep.

   3. the baby cries.

   4. the uterus becomes firm.

5. A woman had a midline episiotomy performed at delivery. The primary purpose of the episiotomy is to

   1. allow forceps to be applied.

   2. enlarge the vaginal opening.

   3. eliminate the possibility of lacerations.

   4. eliminate the need for cesarean birth.

6. A woman is admitted to the hospital in labor. Vaginal examination reveals that she is 8 cm dilated. At this point in her labor, which of the following statements would the nurse expect her to make?

   1. "I can't decide what to name my baby."

   2. "It feels good to push with each contraction."

   3. "Take your hand off my stomach when I have a contraction."

   4. "This isn't as bad as I expected."

7. The nurse is caring for a woman who is in labor. She is 8 cm dilated. To support her during this phase of her labor, the nurse should

   1. leave her alone most of the time.

   2. offer her a back rub during contractions.

   3. offer her sips of oral fluids.

   4. provide her with warm blankets.

8. A woman in labor is placed on an external fetal monitor. The nurse notices that the fetal heart rate is erratic during contractions but returns to baseline at the end of each contraction. This should be recorded as

   1. early decelerations.
   2. variable decelerations.
   3. late decelerations.
   4. fetal distress.

9. During labor, the nurse observes variable decelerations on the external fetal monitor. The best action for the nurse to take at this time is to

   1. apply an oxygen mask.
   2. change the woman's position to left side-lying.
   3. get the woman out of bed and walk her around.
   4. move the woman to the delivery room.

10. During delivery, a mediolateral episiotomy is performed and a 7 lb 8 oz baby delivered. Which of the following nursing assessments indicate a postpartum complication and are not normal? Check all that apply.

    _____ A foul lochial odor.

    _____ Discomfort while sitting.

    _____ Ecchymosis and edema of the perineum.

    _____ Separation of the episiotomy wound edges.

11. The nurse is talking with a woman who is 36 weeks' gestation during a prenatal visit. Which statement indicates that the woman understands the onset of labor?

    1. "I need to go to the hospital as soon as the contractions become painful."
    2. "If I experience bright red vaginal bleeding I know that I am about to deliver."
    3. "I need to go to the hospital when I am having regular contractions and bloody show."
    4. "My labor will not start until after my membranes rupture and I gush fluid."

12. Using Leopold's maneuvers to determine fetal position, the nurse finds that the fetus is in a vertex position with the back on the left side. Where is the best place for the nurse to listen for fetal heart tones?

    1. In the right upper quadrant of the mother's abdomen.
    2. In the left upper quadrant of the mother's abdomen.
    3. In the right lower quadrant of the mother's abdomen.
    4. In the left lower quadrant of the mother's abdomen.

13. Which of the following is the best way for the nurse to assess contractions in a client presenting to the labor and delivery area?

    1. Place the client on the electronic fetal monitor with the labor toco at the fundus.

    2. Ask the client to describe the frequency, duration, and strength of her contractions.

    3. Use Leopold's maneuvers to determine the quality of the uterine contractions.

    4. Place the fingertips of one hand on the fundus to determine frequency, duration, and strength of contractions.

14. As the nurse assigned to a laboring woman, you are observing the fetal heart rate. Which of the following findings would you consider abnormal for a client in active labor?

    1. A rate of 160 with no significant changes through a contraction.

    2. A rate of 130 with accelerations to 150 with fetal movement.

    3. A rate that varies between 120 and 130.

    4. A rate of 170 with a drop to 140 during a contraction.

15. A woman arrives at the birthing center in active labor. On examination, the cervix is 5 cm dilated, membranes intact and bulging, and the presenting part at −1 station. The woman asks if she can go for a walk. What is the best response for the nurse to give?

    1. "I think it would be best for you to remain in bed at this time because of the risk of cord prolapse."

    2. "It's fine for you to walk, but please stay nearby. If you feel a gush of fluid, I will need to check you and your baby."

    3. "It will be fine for you to walk because that will assist the natural body forces to bring the baby down the birth canal."

    4. "I would be glad to get you a bean bag chair or rocker instead."

16. A primigravida presents to the labor room with rupture of membranes at 40 weeks' gestation. Her cervix is 2 cm dilated and 100% effaced. Contractions are every 10 minutes. What should the nurse include in the plan of care?

    1. Allow her to ambulate as desired as long as the presenting part is engaged.

    2. Assess fetal heart tones and maternal status every five minutes.

    3. Place her on an electronic fetal monitor for continuous assessment of labor.

    4. Send her home with instructions to return when contractions are every 5 minutes.

17. A woman who is in active labor at 4 cm dilated, 100% effaced, and 0 station is ambulating and experiences a gush of fluid. What is the most appropriate initial action for the nurse to take?

   1. Send a specimen of the amniotic fluid to the laboratory for analysis.

   2. Have the woman return to her room and place her in Trendelenburg position to prevent cord prolapse.

   3. Have the woman return to her room so that you can assess fetal status, including auscultation of fetal heart tones for one full minute.

   4. Call the woman's physician because a cesarean delivery will be required.

18. The nurse is providing care to a woman. During the most recent vaginal examination the nurse feels the cervix 6 cm dilated, 100% effaced, with the vertex at −1 station. What is the best interpretation of this information? The woman is in

   1. active labor with the head as presenting part not yet engaged.

   2. transition with the backside as presenting part fully engaged.

   3. latent phase labor with the backside as presenting part fully engaged.

   4. active labor with the head as presenting part fully engaged.

19. A woman is completely dilated and at +2 station. Her contractions are strong and last 50–70 seconds. Based on this information, the nurse should know that the client is in which stage of labor?

   1. First stage.

   2. Second stage.

   3. Third stage.

   4. Fourth stage.

20. A 28-year-old primigravida is admitted to the labor room. She is 2 cm dilated, 90% effaced, and the head is at 0 station. Contractions are every 10 minutes lasting 20–30 seconds. Membranes are intact. Admitting vital signs are: blood pressure 110/70, pulse 78, respirations 16, temperature 98.8° F, and fetal heart rate 144. The nurse plans to monitor

   1. blood pressure and contractions hourly and fetal heart rate every 15 minutes.

   2. temperature, blood pressure, and contractions every 4 hours and fetal heart rate hourly.

   3. contractions, effacement, and dilation of cervix, and fetal heart rate every hour.

   4. contractions, blood pressure, and fetal heart rate every 15 minutes.

21. A woman's cervix is completely dilated with the head at -2 station. The head has not descended in the past hour. What is the most appropriate initial assessment for the nurse to make?

    1. Assess to determine if the client's bladder is distended.

    2. Send the client for X-rays to determine fetal size.

    3. Notify the surgical team so that an operative delivery can be planned.

    4. Assess fetal status, including fetal heart tones, and scalp pH.

22. A woman who has been in labor for 6 hours is now 9 cm dilated and has intense contractions every 1 to 2 minutes. She is anxious and feels the need to bear down with her contractions. What is the best action for the nurse to take?

    1. Allow her to push so that delivery can be expedited.

    2. Encourage panting breathing through contractions to prevent pushing.

    3. Reposition her in a squatting position to make her more comfortable.

    4. Provide back rubs during contractions to distract her.

23. A newborn, at 1 minute after vaginal delivery, is pink with blue hands and feet, has a lusty cry, heart rate 140, prompt response to stimulation with crying, and maintains minimal flexion, with sluggish movement. The nurse should know that this newborn's Apgar score is

    1. 10.

    2. 9.

    3. 8.

    4. 7.

24. A woman delivered a 7 lb boy by spontaneous vaginal delivery 30 minutes ago. Her fundus is firm at the umbilicus and she has moderate lochia rubra. Which nursing diagnosis is highest priority as the nurse plans care?

    1. Risk for infection related to episiotomy.

    2. Constipation related to fear of pain.

    3. Potential for impaired urinary elimination related to perineal edema.

    4. Deficient knowledge related to lack of knowledge regarding newborn care.

25. A woman is in the fourth stage of labor. She and her new daughter are together in the room. What assessments are essential for the nurse to make during this time?

    1. Assess the pattern and frequency of contractions and the infant's vital signs.

    2. Assess the woman's vital signs, fundus, bladder, perineal condition, and lochia. Assess the infant's vital signs.

3. Assess the woman's vital signs, fundus, bladder, perineal condition, and lochia. Return the infant to the nursery.

4. Assess the infant for obvious abnormalities. Assess the woman for blood loss and firm uterine contraction.

26. A woman, G3 P2, was admitted at 32 weeks' gestation contracting every 7-10 minutes. Her cervix is 2 cm dilated and 70% effaced. What should the nurse include in the plan of care for this client?

    1. Discuss with the client the need to stop working after her discharge from the hospital.

    2. Monitor the client and her fetus for response to impending delivery.

    3. Assess the client's past pregnancy history to determine if she has experienced preterm labor in the past.

    4. Start oral terbutaline to stop the contractions.

27. A woman was admitted in premature labor contracting every 5 minutes. Her cervix is 3 cm dilated and 100% effaced, IV magnesium sulfate at 1 g per hour is infusing. How will the nurse know the drug is having the desired effect?

    1. The contractions will increase in frequency to every 3 minutes, although there will be no further cervical changes.

    2. The woman will be able to sleep through her contractions due to the sedative effect of the magnesium sulfate.

    3. The contractions will diminish in frequency and finally disappear.

    4. The woman will have diminished deep tendon reflexes and her blood pressure will decrease.

28. A woman has just received an epidural for anesthesia during her labor. What should the nurse include in the plan of care because of the anesthesia?

    1. Assist the client in position changes and observe for signs of labor progress.

    2. Administer 500-1000 ml of a sugar-free crystalloid solution.

    3. Place a Foley catheter as soon as the anesthesia has been administered.

    4. Offer the client a back rub to reduce the discomfort of her contractions.

29. A woman delivered her infant son 3 hours ago. She had an episiotomy to facilitate delivery. As the nurse assigned to care for her, which of the following would be the most appropriate action?

1. Place an ice pack on the perineum.
2. Apply a heat lamp to the perineum.
3. Take her for a sitz bath.
4. Administer analgesic medication as ordered.

30. A woman is scheduled for a cesarean section delivery due to a transverse fetal lie. What is the best way for the nurse to evaluate that she understands the procedure?

    1. Ask her about the help she will have at home after her delivery.
    2. Give her a diagram of the body and ask her to draw the procedure for you.
    3. Ask her to tell you what she knows about the scheduled surgery.
    4. Provide her with a booklet explaining cesarean deliveries when she arrives at the hospital.

ANSWERS AND RATIONALES

1. 4. Gastric motility is decreased during pregnancy. Food eaten several hours prior to the onset of labor may still be in the stomach undigested. This will influence the type of anesthesia the client may receive.

2. 2. With the baby in a vertex, LOA presentation and no other indicators of distress, amniotic fluid should be clear to straw-colored.

3. 3. Immediately after the rupture of membranes, the fetal heart tones are checked, then checked again after the next contraction or after 5-10 minutes.

4. 4. Oxytoxic medications such as Pitocin, Methergine, and Ergotrate are administered to stimulate uterine contractility and reverse fundal relaxation in the postdelivery client.

5. 2. An episiotomy is an incision made in the perineum to enlarge the vaginal opening, allowing additional room for the birth of the baby.

6. 3. At 8 cm dilated the client is in the transition stage of her labor. Many women experience hyperesthesia of the skin at this time and would not want to be touched during a contraction.

7. 2. The counterpressure of a back rub during a contraction may relieve discomfort.

8. 2. Variable decelerations are frequently caused by transient fetal pressure on the cord and are not a sign of fetal distress. A change in the mother's position will usually relieve the problem.

9. 2. Changing the position of the mother will relieve transient pressure on the umbilical cord.

10. *A foul lochial odor* should be checked. This is a sign of infection.
    Ecchymosis and edema of the perineum should be checked. This could be caused by a number of things but indicates recovery will be prolonged.
    Separation of the episiotomy wound edges should be checked. This might be due to infection or trauma. In this case the episiotomy wound would have to heal by second intention (wound left open to heal) or third intention (wound resutured).

11. 3. Regular contractions coupled with bloody show suggest that cervical changes are occurring as a result of contractions.

12. 4. The left lower quadrant is the correct location since the back is on the left and the vertex is in the pelvis.

13. 4. The fingertips of one hand allow the nurse to feel when the contraction begins and ends and to determine the strength of the construction by the firmness of the uterus.

14. 4. A rate of 170 is suggestive of fetal tachycardia. A drop to 140 during a contraction represents some periodic change, which is not a normal finding.

15. 2. Although there is always some risk of complications when membranes rupture, it is safe for this woman to ambulate as long as she is rechecked if rupture of membranes occurs.

16. 1. Ambulation will help contractions more effectively dilate the cervix. As long as the presenting part is engaged, there is no increased risk of cord prolapse.

17. 3. The most important nursing action after rupture of the membranes is careful fetal assessment, including fetal heart tones counted for 1 minute.

18. 1. At 6 cm dilation and complete effacement, active labor is occurring. A station of -1 indicates that the vertex is above the ischial spines and not fully engaged.

19. 2. The second stage of labor extends from complete cervical dilation to delivery of the infant.

20. 1. During early labor, blood pressure and contractions should be monitored hourly and fetal heart rate every 15 minutes.

21. 1. A full bladder may prevent the head from moving down into the pelvic inlet. Often clients do not have the sensation of a full bladder late in labor, despite significant distention.

22. 2. Since the client is still in transition and not ready to deliver, encouraging her to pant will diminish the urge to push.

23. 3. This infant has 2 points for heart rate, respiratory effort, and reflex irritability. One point is awarded for color and muscle tone for a total of 8.

24. 3. Perineal edema may affect urinary elimination. If allowed to continue, it may also lead to excessive postpartum bleeding because the uterus cannot stay firmly contracted when the bladder is excessively full.

25. 2. Assessment of the mother during fourth stage includes elements related to her recovery from childbirth. Infant assessment focuses on stability and transition to extrauterine life.

26. 3. As a G3 P2, the client's past pregnancy history may provide some important information that may shape the care rendered at this time.

27. 3. If the magnesium sulfate is effective you would expect the contractions to decrease and then disappear. You would not continue to perform vaginal exams if the desired result is occurring.

28. 1. Epidural anesthesia may diminish the client's sensation of painful stimuli and movement. Assistance and frequent assessment are therefore essential.

29. 1. Ice during the first 12 hours after delivery causes vasoconstriction and thereby prevents edema. Ice also provides pain relief through numbing of the area.

30. 3. Asking for clarification of what she knows is the best way to evaluate what she understands of the procedure. If the client has additional questions, the nurse can then clarify or amplify the information.

5

The Postpartum Period

■ OVERVIEW

Physical Changes of the Postpartum Period

A. The postpartum period is defined as that period of time, usually 6 weeks, in which the mother's body experiences anatomic and physiologic changes that reverse the body's adaptation to pregnancy; may also be called *involution*.

CHAPTER OUTLINE

Overview

Postpartal Psychosocial Changes

Assessment

Analysis

Planning and Implementation

Evaluation

Complications of the Postpartum Period

B. Begins with the delivery of the placenta and ends when all body systems are returned to, or nearly to, their prepregnant state.

C. May or may not include the return of the ovulatory/menstrual cycle.

Specific Body System Changes

Reproductive System

A. Uterus undergoes involution—return to prepregnant size and position in pelvis.

    1. Fundus palpated at the umbilicus in midline at 1 hour postpartum.

    2. Fundus may rise up to 1 cm above umbilicus within 12 hours then begin descent of 1 cm per day until no longer palpable by day 10.

    3. The endometrial surface is sloughed off as *lochia*, in three stages

        a. *Lochia rubra*: red color, days 1-3 after delivery; consists of blood and cellular debris from decidua.

        b. *Lochia serosa*: pinkish brown, days 4-10; mostly serum, some blood, tissue debris.

        c. *Lochia alba*: yellowish white, days 11-21 up to 6 weeks; mostly leukocytes, with decidua, epithelial cells, mucus.

    4. Lochia has a particular, musty odor. Foul-smelling lochia, however, may indicate infection. Some small dark clots may be normal immediately after delivery; large clots and bright red clots signify the need for close investigation.

  5. The placental site heals by means of exfoliative shedding,
      a process that allows the upward growth of the new
      endometrium and the prevention of scar tissue at the
      old placental site. This process may take
      six weeks.
B. Cervix
  1. Flabby immediately after delivery; closes slowly.
  2. Admits one fingertip by the end of one week after delivery.
  3. Shape of external os changed by delivery from round to slitlike
      opening
C. Vagina
  1. Edematous after delivery
  2. May have small lacerations
  3. Smooth-walled for 3-4 weeks, then rugae reappear
  4. Hypoestrogenic until ovulation and menstruation resume
D. Ovulation/menstruation
  1. First cycle is usually anovulatory.
  2. If not lactating, menses may resume in 6-8 weeks.
  3. If lactating, menses less predictable; may resume
      in 12-24 weeks.
E. Breasts
  1. Nonlactating woman
      a. Prolactin levels fall rapidly.
      b. May still secrete colostrum for 2-3 days.
      c. Engorgement of breast tissue resulting from temporary congestion
          of veins and lymphatic circulation occurs on third day, lasts
          24-36 hours, usually resolves spontaneously.
      d. Client should wear tight bra to compress ducts and use cold
          applications to reduce swelling.
  2. Lactating woman
      a. High level of prolactin immediately after delivery of placenta
          continued by frequent contact with nursing baby.
      b. Initial secretion is colostrum, with increasing amounts of true
          breast milk appearing between 48-96 hours.
      c. Milk "let-down" reflex caused by oxytocin from posterior pituitary
          released by sucking.
      d. Successful lactation results from the complex interaction of infant
          sucking reflexes and the maternal production and let-down of
          milk.

Abdominal Wall/Skin

A. Muscles relaxed, separation of the rectus muscle (diastasis recti) from 2 to
    4 cm, usually resolves by 6 weeks with exercise.
B. Stretch marks gradually fade to silvery-white appearance.

Cardiovascular System

A. Normal blood loss in delivery of single infant is less than 500 cc (up to 1000 cc normal blood loss for a c-section).
B. Hematocrit usually returns to prepregnancy value within 4-6 weeks.
C. WBC count increases up to 20,000.
D. Increased clotting factors remain for several weeks leaving woman at risk for problems with thrombi.
E. Varicosities regress.

Urinary System

A. May have difficulty voiding in immediate postpartum period as a result of urethral edema and lack of sensation.
B. Marked diuresis begins within 12 hours of delivery; increases volume of urinary output as well as perspiration loss.
C. Lactosuria may be seen in nursing mothers.
D. Many women will show slight proteinuria during first 1-2 days of involution.

Gastrointestinal System

A. Mother usually hungry after delivery; good appetite is expected.
B. May still experience constipation from lack of muscle tone in abdomen and intestinal tract, and perineal soreness.

Other

All other systems experience normal and rapid regression to prepregnancy status.

■ POSTPARTAL PSYCHOSOCIAL CHANGES

Adaptation to Parenthood

Motor Skills

New parents must learn new physical skills to care for infant (e.g., feeding, holding, burping, changing diapers, skin care).

Attachment Skills

A. *Bonding*: the development of a caring relationship with the baby. Behaviors include
   1. Claiming: identifying the ways in which the baby looks or acts like members of the family.
   2. Identification: establishing the baby's unique nature (assigning the baby his or her own name).
   3. Attachment is facilitated by positive feedback between baby and caregivers.

B. Sensual responses enhance adaptation to parenthood.
   1. Touch: from fingertip, to open palm, to enfolding; touch is an important communication with the baby.
   2. Eye-to-eye contact: a cultural activity that helps to form a trusting relationship.
   3. Voice: parents await the baby's first cry; babies respond to the higher-pitched voice that parents use in talking to the baby.
   4. Odor: babies quickly identify their own mother's breast milk by odor.
   5. Entrainment: babies move in rhythm to patterns of adult speech.
   6. Biorhythm: babies respond to maternal heartbeats.

Maternal Adjustment

Takes place in three phases.

Dependent/"Taking In"

A. 1–2 days after delivery.
B. Mother's needs predominate; mother passive and dependent.
C. Mother needs to talk about labor and delivery experiences to integrate them into the fabric of her life.
D. Mother may need help with everyday activities, as well as child care.
E. Food/sleep important.

Dependent/Independent/"Taking Hold"

A. By third day mother begins to reassert herself.
B. Identifies own needs, especially for teaching and help with her own and baby's needs.
C. Some emotional lability, may cry "for no reason."
D. Mother requires reassurance that she can perform tasks of motherhood.

Independent/"Letting Go"

A. Usually evident by fifth or sixth week.
B. Shows pattern of lifestyle that includes new baby but still focuses on entire family as unit.
C. Reestablishment of father-mother bond seen in this period.
D. Mother may still feel tired and overwhelmed by responsibility and conflicting demands on her time and energies.

■ ASSESSMENT

Physical

A. Vital signs
   1. Individual protocol until stable, then at least once every 8 hours.

DELEGATION TIP

Vital signs assessment may be delegated to ancillary personnel. Instruct personnel to report an oral temperature over 100.4°F after the first 24 hours postpartum or to report the presence of chills.

   2. Temperature over 100.4°F (37.8°C) after first 24 hours, lasting more than 48 hours, indicative of infection.
B. Fundus
   1. Assessment done with empty bladder, one hand supporting base of uterus and one on fundus
   2. Assess for firmness and position
C. Lochia: color, amount, clots, odor
D. Perineum
   1. Healing of episiotomy
   2. Hematoma formation
   3. Development of hemorrhoids
E. Breasts: firmness, condition of nipples
F. Elimination patterns: voiding, flatus, bowels
G. Legs: pain, warmth, tenderness indicating thrombosis
H. Perform foot dorsiflexion (Homan's sign)

Psychosocial Adjustment
A. Overall emotional status of parents
B. Parents' knowledge of infant needs
C. Previous experience of parents
D. Physical condition of infant
E. Ethnocultural background and financial status of parents
F. Additional family support available to parents

◼ ANALYSIS
Nursing diagnoses for the postpartum period may include
A. Risk for constipation
B. Deficient knowledge
C. Self-care deficit
D. Impaired urinary elimination
E. Interrupted family process
F. Risk for impaired parenting
G. Ineffective role performance
H. Pain

■ PLANNING AND IMPLEMENTATION
Goals

A. Involution and return to prepregnancy state will be accomplished without complication.
B. Parental role(s) will be successfully assumed.
C. New baby will be successfully integrated into family structure.
D. Successful infant feeding patterns (bottle- or breastfeeding) will be established

Interventions
Physical Care

A. Assess mother according to individual needs during first critical hours after delivery; implement nursing interventions as needed.
B. Implement routine postpartum care after first hours.
   1. Administer medications as ordered (e.g., oxytocins, analgesics).
   2. Teach perineal care.
   3. Perform other care as needed (e.g., heat, cold applications).
   4. Measure first voiding for sufficiency, observe I&O for first 24 hours.
   5. Assist with breastfeeding as needed.
   6. Instruct in breast care for bottle-feeding mother—good bra, limiting nipple stimulation.
C. Encourage measures to promote bowel function: roughage in diet, ambulation, sufficient fluids, attention to urge to defecate. Reassure about integrity of episiotomy.

Adjustment to Parenthood

A. Provide time for parents to be alone with baby in crucial early time after delivery.
B. Identify learning needs of parents.
C. Plan teaching to include both parents where possible.
D. Help parents realize that fatigue is normal at this time.
E. Help parents identify and strengthen their own coping mechanisms.
F. Help parents identify resources available to them.
G. Promote positive self-esteem on part of parents as they learn new role(s).
H. Provide anticipatory guidance for after discharge.
I. Provide information about contraception if requested.
J. Prepare for discharge: reinforce physician's instructions about activities, rest, diet, drugs, exercise, resumption of sexual intercourse, return for postpartum examination.

Infant Feeding

A. General information

CLIENT TEACHING CHECKLIST

Encourage a fluid intake of 2000 ml/day to promote successful infant feeding.

1. Infancy is a time of rapid growth and development; infant doubles birth weight in 4–6 months, triples birth weight by 1 year.
2. Newborns lose up to 8% of their birth weight, then gain 4–7 ounces per week.

B. Choices in newborn nutrition
   1. Breastfeeding: optimal infant nutrition, easily digested, contains antibodies to bolster the immune system as well as all nutrients needed by the infant.
      a. Helps mother's body return to prepregnant state faster.
      b. Provides some child-spacing but should not be relied on.
      c. Prolactin, stimulated by the infant's sucking, stimulates milk production.
      d. Oxytocin causes "let-down" or delivery of milk to nursing baby.
   2. Formula-feeding (bottle-feeding): utilizes modified cow's milk or soy formulas as basis for provision of 20 kcal/oz.
      a. Formulas are widely available in ready-to-feed, concentrated, and powdered forms.
      b. They have supplemental vitamins; may also contain added iron.
      c. Concentrated and powdered forms require addition of prescribed amounts of water for appropriate reconstitution.
      d. Bottles and nipples should be carefully cleaned daily by hand and rinsed with boiling water or by electric dishwasher.
      e. Powdered or concentrated formulas should be mixed with boiled water.

C. Nursing measures to promote successful infant feeding
   1. Assess previous experience and knowledge of process of infant feeding.
   2. Demonstrate how to hold baby for breastfeeding and for feeding with formula.
   3. Show how to burp baby.
   4. Allow time for practice with selected feeding method.
   5. Provide positive reinforcement for successful actions.
   6. Give written instructions for at-home reference.
   7. Help parents identify progress and pleasure in feeding infant.
   8. If bottle-feeding, demonstrate how to prepare formula using appropriate method.
   9. If breastfeeding, assess breasts for tenderness or discomfort, and examine nipples for cracks, bleeding, soreness, and erectility.

NURSING ALERT

Recognize differences in cultural practices among breastfeeding women:

- North American and European: resistance to breast exposure; considered indecent.
- Muslim women are encouraged to breast feed children until they are two years of age.
- Hispanic women do not offer colostrum to the newborn.

10. Assist mother with preparation: clean hands, comfortable position, support as needed (extra pillows). Demonstrate alternate infant positioning, e.g., "football hold."
11. Bring infant to nurse as soon as possible after delivery.
12. Demonstrate positioning of baby at breast, initiate rooting reflex, place entire nipple and as much of areola as possible into baby's mouth, depress fleshy part of breast away from baby's nose if needed.
13. Allow baby to nurse in short frequent periods, lengthening gradually in later days. Alternate breast offered first.
14. Help mother release baby from nipple by breaking suction of baby on nipple. Check for nipple trauma.
15. Help mother move baby to alternate breast if needed.
16. Remain with mother at each feeding until she feels confident: see also Table 5-1 for additional information on breastfeeding.
17. Assist bottle-feeding mother with suppression of lactation, accomplished primarily by mechanical inhibition.
   a. Mechanical inhibition: usually takes 48–72 hours
      1) snug breast binder for 2–3 days postdelivery
      2) applications of cold (ice packs) and analgesia to relieve discomfort
      3) avoidance of heat or other stimuli to breasts that increase milk production (including breast pumps)
      4) a well-fitting bra until lactation is suppressed
   b. No approved medications to suppress lactation.

■ EVALUATION

A. Involution successfully initiated and progressing without complication
B. Parents begin to assume new role behaviors and identities
C. Beginning integration of newborn into family structure; bonding established
D. Infant feeding techniques mastered; infant growing and developing appropriately

TABLE 5-1   Tips for Successful Breastfeeding

Breast care	Do not use soap on nipples or areola. Expose nipples to air to toughen them. Know how to pump breast milk if necessary and how to store expressed breast milk.
Nutrition	Need for good maternal nutrition while nursing. • Additional 300–600 kcal/day • 2–3 liters fluid/day Know that certain foods may make the baby fussy and will need to be avoided temporarily.
Comfort	Wear well-fitting bra; use absorbent pads without plastic coating if leaking occurs. Uterine cramping during nursing normal at first.
Medications	Avoid medications excreted in breast milk (mother should check with physician before taking any drug while nursing). Birth control pills should not be taken while nursing (decreases milk production).
Sources of help	Inform mother of community support groups available for nursing mothers.

E. Parents comfortable about infant care techniques and can demonstrate knowledge

Teaching: Postpartum/Discharge

A. Postpartum
1. Normal events of postpartum period: physical, psychosocial
2. Information about feeding her infant
3. Basic infant care, including cord care, bathing, circumcision care, dressing, handling, signs of illness
4. Safety needs of infant
5. Recommendations concerning activities
6. Specific teaching about any medications

B. Discharge
1. Reinforcement of all postpartum teaching, allowing parent(s) time to ask questions.
2. Referrals to professional assistance (MD, CNM, hospital's maternity unit, etc.).
3. Referrals to appropriate community assistance groups (Nursing Mothers, Mothers of Twins, etc.) that meet individual needs.
4. Scheduled appointments for postpartal examination/newborn's first well-baby examination.

5. Literature to reinforce all teaching. Excitement and anxiety of discharge may interfere with learning; literature will be available for quick reference.

■ COMPLICATIONS OF THE POSTPARTUM PERIOD

Postpartum Hemorrhage

A. General information
   1. Major cause of maternal death
   2. Loss of more than 500 ml blood at the time of delivery or immediately thereafter is considered postpartum hemorrhage.
   3. Major causes include
      a. Uterine atony: loss of muscle tone in the uterus; may be the result of overdistension (large baby, multiple pregnancy, polyhydramnios), overmassage, maternal exhaustion, inhalation anesthesia
      b. Laceration of the birth canal (cervix, vagina, labia, perineum)
      c. Retained placental fragments or incomplete expulsion of placenta (usually the cause of late postpartum hemorrhage)
      d. Placenta accreta: penetration of the myometrium by the trophoblast, resulting in abnormal adherence of the placenta to the uterine wall. Rare; requires manual removal of the placenta
B. Assessment findings
   1. "Boggy" uterus, relaxed state indicating atony
   2. If uterus is firm with excess bleeding, may indicate lacerations.
   3. Bright red blood, with clots
      a. Large amounts with atony
      b. Steady trickle with lacerations
   4. Hemorrhage immediately after delivery with atony or lacerations
   5. With retained placental fragments, delay of up to 2 weeks
   6. With severe blood loss, signs and symptoms of shock
   7. Full bladder may displace uterus and prevent it from contracting firmly.
C. Nursing interventions
   1. Identify clients at risk for bleeding.
   2. Monitor fundus frequently if bleeding occurs; when stable, every 15 minutes for 1-2 hours, then at appropriate intervals.
   3. Monitor maternal vital signs for indications of shock.
   4. Administer medications, IV fluids as ordered.
   5. Measure I&O.
   6. Remain with client for support and explanation of procedures.
   7. Keep client warm.
   8. Prepare for client's transfer to surgery if needed for repair of laceration or removal of placental fragment.
   9. Monitor for signs of DIC.

Thrombophlebitis

A. General information
  1. Formation of a thrombus when a vein wall is inflamed
  2. May be seen in the veins of the legs or pelvis
  3. May result from injury, infection, or the normal increase in circulating clotting factors in the pregnant and newly delivered woman.
B. Assessment findings
  1. Pain/discomfort in area of thrombus (legs, pelvis, abdomen)
  2. If in the leg, pain, edema, redness over affected area
  3. Elevated temperature and chills
  4. Peripheral pulses may be decreased
  5. Positive Homan's sign
  6. If in a deep vein, leg may be cool and pale
C. Nursing interventions
  1. Maintain bed rest with leg elevated on pillow. Never raise knee gatch on bed.
  2. Apply moist heat as ordered.
  3. Administer analgesics as ordered.
  4. Provide bed cradle to keep sheets off leg.
  5. Administer anticoagulant therapy as ordered (usually heparin), and observe client for signs of bleeding.
  6. Apply elastic support hose if ordered, with daily inspection of legs with hose removed.
  7. Teach client *not* to massage legs.
  8. Allow client to express fears and reactions to condition.
  9. Observe client for signs of pulmonary embolism.
  10. Continue to bring baby to mother for feeding and interaction.

Subinvolution

A. General information
  1. Failure of the uterus to revert to prepregnant state through gradual reduction in size and placement
  2. May be caused by infection, retained placental fragments, or tumors in the uterus
B. Assessment findings
  1. Uterus remains enlarged
  2. Fundus higher in the abdomen than anticipated
  3. Lochia does not progress from rubra to serosa to alba
  4. If caused by infection, possible leukorrhea and backache
C. Nursing interventions
  1. Teach client to recognize unusual bleeding patterns.
  2. Teach client usual pattern of uterine involution.
  3. Instruct client to report abnormal bleeding to physician.
  4. Administer oxytoxic medications if ordered.

Postpartum Infection

A. General information
   1. Any infection of the reproductive tract, associated with giving birth, usually occurring within 10 days of the birth
   2. Predisposing factors include
      a. Prolonged rupture of membranes
      b. Cesarean birth
      c. Trauma during birth process
      d. Maternal anemia
      e. Retained placental fragments
   3. Infection may be localized or systemic
B. Assessment findings
   1. Temperature of 100.4°F (37.8°C) or more for 2 consecutive days, excluding the first 24 hours
   2. Abdominal, perineal, or pelvic pain
   3. Foul-smelling vaginal discharge
   4. Burning sensation with urination
   5. Chills, malaise
   6. Rapid pulse and respirations
   7. Elevated WBC count (may be normal for postpartum initially), positive culture/sensitivity report for causative organism
C. Nursing interventions
   1. Force fluids: client may need more than 3 liters/day.
   2. Administer antibiotics and other medications as ordered.
   3. Treat symptoms as they arise (e.g., warm sitz bath for infection in episiotomy).
   4. Encourage high-calorie, high-protein diet to promote tissue healing.
   5. Position client in semi- to high-Fowler's to promote drainage and prevent reflux higher into reproductive tract.
   6. Support mother if isolated from baby.

Mastitis

A. General information
   1. Infection of the breast, usually unilateral
   2. Frequently caused by cracked nipples in the nursing mother
   3. Causative organism usually hemolytic *S. aureus*
   4. If untreated, may result in breast abscess.
B. Assessment findings
   1. Redness, tenderness, or hardened area in the breast
   2. Maternal chills, malaise
   3. Elevated vital signs, especially temperature and pulse
C. Nursing interventions
   1. Teach/stress importance of hand washing to nursing mother, and wash own hands before touching client's breast.

2. Administer antibiotics as ordered.
3. Apply ice if ordered between feedings.
4. Empty breast regularly: baby may continue to nurse or have mother use hospital-grade pump.

Urinary Tract Infection

A. General information: may be caused postpartally by coliform bacteria, coupled with bladder trauma during the delivery, or a break in technique during catheterization.
B. Assessment findings
   1. Pain in the suprapubic area or at the costovertebral angle
   2. Fever
   3. Burning, urgency, frequency on urination
   4. Increased WBC count and hematuria
   5. Urine culture positive for causative organism
C. Nursing interventions
   1. Check status of bladder frequently in postpartum client.
   2. Use nursing measures to encourage client to void.
   3. Force fluids: may need minimum of 3 liters/day.
   4. Catheterize client if ordered, using sterile technique.
   5. Administer medications as ordered.
   6. Monitor status of progress through continuing lab tests.
   7. Support mother with explanations of interventions.
   8. No need for baby to be separated from mother.

REVIEW QUESTIONS

1. On the second day postpartum, the nurse asks the new mother to describe her vaginal bleeding. The nurse should expect her to say that it is
   1. red and moderate.
   2. red with clots.
   3. scant and brown.
   4. thin and white.

2. A woman delivers a 6 lb 4 oz (2835 g) baby boy. Which of the following statements would indicate to the nurse that the mother has begun to integrate her new baby into the family structure?
   1. "All this baby does is cry. He's not like my other child."
   2. "I wish he had curly hair like my husband."
   3. "My parents wanted a granddaughter."
   4. "When he yawns, he looks just like his brother."

3. A diabetic woman plans to breastfeed her baby. The nurse explains that, if she is hyperglycemic,
   1. the glucose content of her breast milk may be high.
   2. the production of milk may be impaired.
   3. her baby will receive insulin in the milk.
   4. her baby will not grow well.

4. A woman and her roommate each delivered a child 2 days ago. One is breastfeeding; one is using formula. Which of the following instructions can the nurse give to both mothers?
   1. Wear a good, well-supporting bra.
   2. Apply warm compresses to breast if too full.
   3. Apply cold compresses to breast if too full.
   4. Do not apply any soap to your nipples.

5. Because this is a woman's third child, the nurse should not be surprised if she complains of
   1. chest pain.
   2. afterbirth cramps.
   3. burning on urination.
   4. chills.

6. A woman delivered a male infant yesterday. While caring for her on her first postpartum day, which of the following behaviors would you expect?
   1. Asking specific questions about home care of the infant.
   2. Concern about when her bowels will move.
   3. Frequent crying spells for unexplained reasons.
   4. Acceptance of the nurse's suggestions about personal care.

7. A woman delivered this morning. Because this is her first child, which of the following goals is most appropriate?
   1. Early discharge for mother and baby.
   2. Rapid adaptation to role of parent.
   3. Effective education of both parents.
   4. Minimal need for expression of negative feelings.

8. A new mother is going to breastfeed her baby. What is the best indication that the let-down reflex has been achieved in a nursing mother?
   1. Increased prolactin levels.
   2. Milk dripping from the opposite breast.

3. Progressive weight gain in the infant.

4. Relief of breast engorgement.

9. To prevent cracked nipples while she is breastfeeding, the mother should be taught to

   1. apply lanolin prior to feedings.

   2. nurse at least 20 minutes on each breast the first day.

   3. use plastic bra liners.

   4. wash her nipples with water only.

10. What is the best indication that the breastfed baby is digesting the breast milk properly?

    1. The baby does not experience colic.

    2. The baby passes dark green, pasty stools.

    3. The baby passes soft, golden-yellow stools.

    4. The baby sleeps for several hours after each feeding.

11. Which of the following observations in the postpartum period would be of most concern to the nurse?

    1. After delivery, the mother touches the newborn with her fingertips.

    2. The new parents asked the nurse to recommend a good baby care book.

    3. A new father holds his son in the en face position while visiting.

    4. A new mother sits in bed while her newborn lies awake in the crib.

12. A woman has just delivered her first baby who will be breastfed. The nurse should include which of the following instructions in the teaching plan?

    1. Try to schedule feedings at least every three to four hours.

    2. Wash nipples with soap and water before each feeding.

    3. Avoid nursing bras with plastic lining.

    4. Supplement with water between feedings when necessary.

13. A woman's prenatal antibody titer shows that she is not immune to rubella and will receive the immunization after delivery. The nurse would include which of the following instructions in the teaching plan?

    1. Pregnancy must be avoided for the next three months.

    2. Another immunization should be administered in the next pregnancy.

    3. Breastfeeding should be postponed for 5 days after the injection.

    4. An injection will be needed after each succeeding pregnancy.

14. A woman had a normal vaginal delivery 12 hours ago and is to be discharged from the birthing center. The nurse evaluates that the woman

understands the teaching related to the episiotomy and perineal area when she states,

1. "I know the stitches will be removed at my postpartum clinic visit."

2. "The ice pack should be removed for 10 minutes before replacing it."

3. "The anesthetic spray, then the heat lamp, will help a lot."

4. "The water for the Sitz bath should be warm, about 102–105°F."

15. A new mother is bottle-feeding her newborn. The nurse evaluates that the client understands how to safely manage formula when she states,

1. "Prepared formula should be used within 48 hours."

2. "All bottles, caps, and nipples must be sterilized."

3. "A dishwasher is not sufficient for proper cleaning."

4. "Prepared formula must be refrigerated until used."

16. A woman delivered her baby 12 hours ago. During the postpartum assessment, the uterus is found to be boggy with a heavy lochia flow. The initial action of the nurse is to

1. notify the physician or nurse midwife.

2. administer prn oxytocin.

3. encourage the woman to increase ambulation.

4. massage the uterus until firm.

17. A breastfeeding mother is visited by the home health nurse 2 weeks after delivery. The woman is febrile with flulike symptoms; on assessment the nurse notes a warm, reddened, painful area of the right breast. The best initial action of the nurse is to

1. contact the physician for an order for antibiotics.

2. advise the mother to stop breastfeeding and pumping.

3. assess the mother's feeding technique and knowledge of breast care.

4. obtain a sample of breast milk for culture.

18. A woman had a vaginal delivery of her second child 2 days ago. She is breastfeeding the baby without difficulty. During a postpartum assessment, the nurse would expect the following normal finding.

1. Complaints of afterpains.

2. Pinkish to brownish vaginal discharge.

3. Voiding frequently, 50–75 ml per void.

4. Fundus 1 cm above the umbilicus.

19. A mother who had a vaginal delivery of her first baby 6 weeks ago is seen for her postpartum visit. She is feeling well and is bottle-feeding her infant

successfully. During the physical assessment, the nurse would expect to find the following normal data.

1. Fundus palpated 6 cm below the umbilicus.
2. Breasts tender, some milk expressed.
3. Striae pink but beginning to fade.
4. Creamy, yellow vaginal discharge.

20. A nurse collects the following data on a woman 26 hours after a long labor and a vaginal delivery: temperature 101°F (38.3°C), blood pressure 110/70, pulse 90, some diaphoresis, output 1000 ml per 8 hours, ankle edema, lochia moderate rubra, fundus 1 cm above umbilicus and tender on palpation. The client also asks that the infant be brought back to the nursery. In the analysis of this data, the nurse would select which of the following priority nursing diagnoses?

1. Alteration in parenting related to material discomfort.
2. High risk for injury related to spread of infection.
3. Fluid volume excess related to urinary retention.
4. Knowledge deficit related to uterine subinvolution.

ANSWERS AND RATIONALES

1. 1. Lochia rubra is moderate red discharge and is present for the first 2–3 days postpartum.

2. 4. Family identification of the newborn is an important part of attachment. The first step in identification is defined in terms of likeness to family members.

3. 1. Glucose can be transferred from the serum to the breast, and hyperglycemia may be reflected in the breast milk.

4. 1. A well-fitting, supportive bra with wide straps can be recommended for both the nursing and the nonnursing mother for the support of the breasts and for comfort. The nursing mother's bra should have front flaps over each breast for easy access during nursing.

5. 2. Afterbirth cramps are most common in nursing mothers and multiparas. This mother is both. The release of oxytocin from the posterior pituitary for the "let-down" reflex of lactation causes the afterbirth cramping of the uterus.

6. 4. During the first few days after delivery, the mother is in a dependent phase, initiating little activity by herself, and is usually content to be directed in her activities by a health care provider.

7. 3. Both parents will need education about the new baby—how to care for the baby, information about the baby, and how to be a parent.

8. 2. The nursing infant will stimulate let-down, resulting in milk dripping from the other breast.

9. 4. Nipples should be washed with water only (no soap) to prevent drying.

10. 3. Breastfed babies will pass 6-10 small, loose, yellow stools per day.

11. 4. During the early postpartum period, evidence of maladaptive mothering may include limited handling or smiling at the infant; studies have shown that a predictable group of reciprocal interactions, between mother and baby, should take place with each encounter to foster and reinforce attachment.

12. 3. Although plastic linings protect clothing from leaking milk, the nipples may become sore and prone to infection from trapped moisture; disposable nursing pads can be used to protect clothing.

13. 1. To prevent intrauterine infection, which can result in miscarriage, stillbirth, and congenital rubella syndrome in the fetus, women who are immunized should be advised not to become pregnant for 3 months.

14. 2. To attain the maximum effect of reducing edema and providing numbness of the tissues, the ice pack should remain in place approximately 20 minutes and then be removed for about 10 minutes before replacing it.

15. 4. Extra bottles of prepared formula are stored in the refrigerator and should be warmed slightly before feeding.

16. 4. A soft, boggy uterus should be massaged until firm; clots may be expressed during massage and this often tends to contract the uterus more effectively.

17. 1. These symptoms are signs of infectious mastitis, usually caused by *Staphylococcus aureus; a 10-day course of antibiotics is indicated.*

18. 1. Afterpains occur more commonly in multiparas than in primiparas and are caused by intermittent uterine contractions. Because oxytocin is released when the infant suckles, breastfeeding also increases the severity of the afterpains.

19. 3. At 2 weeks postpartum, striae (stretch marks) are pink and obvious; by 6 weeks they are beginning to fade but may not achieve a silvery appearance for several more weeks.

20. 2. The classic definition of puerperal morbidity resulting from infection is a temperature of 100.4°F (38.0°C) or higher on any of the first 10 days postpartum exclusive of the first 24 hours; additional signs are increased pulse rate, uterine tenderness, foul-smelling lochia, and subinvolution (uterus remains enlarged).

The Newborn

6

■ PHYSIOLOGIC STATUS OF THE NEWBORN

Circulatory

A. Umbilical vein and ductus venosus constrict after cord is clamped; these will become ligaments (2–3 months).

B. Foramen ovale closes functionally as respirations are established, but anatomic or permanent closure may take several months.

C. Ductus arteriosus constricts with establishment of respiratory function; later becomes ligament (2–3 months).

D. Heart rate ranges from 120–160 beats/minute at birth, with changes noted during sleep and activity.

E. Heart murmurs may be heard; usually have little clinical significance.

F. Average blood pressure is 78/42 mmHg.

G. Peripheral circulation established slowly; may have mottled (blue/white) appearance for 24 hours (acrocyanosis).

H. RBC count high immediately after birth, then falls after first week; possible physiologic anemia of infancy.

I. Absence of normal flora in intestine of newborn results in low levels of vitamin K; prophylactic dose of vitamin K given IM on first day of life.

Respiratory

A. "Thoracic squeeze" in vaginal delivery helps drain fluids from respiratory tract; remainder of fluid absorbed across alveolar membranes into capillaries.

B. Adequate levels of surfactants (lecithin and sphingomyelin) ensure mature lung function; prevent alveolar collapse and respiratory distress syndrome.

C. Normal respiratory rate is 30–60 breaths/minute with short periods of apnea (<15 seconds); change noted during sleep or activity.

D. Newborns are obligate nose breathers.

E. Chest and abdomen rise simultaneously; no seesaw breathing.

Renal

A. Urine present in bladder at birth, but newborn may not void for first 12–24 hours; later pattern is 6–10 voidings/day, indicative of sufficient fluid intake.
B. Urine is pale and straw colored; initial voidings may leave brick-red spots on diaper from passage of uric acid crystals in urine.
C. Infant unable to concentrate urine for first 3 months of life.

Digestive

A. Newborn has full cheeks due to well-developed sucking pads.
B. Little saliva is produced.
C. Hard palate should be intact; small raised white areas on palate (*Epstein's pearls*) are normal.
D. Newborn cannot move food from lips to pharynx; nipple needs to be inserted well into mouth.
E. Circumoral pallor may appear while sucking.
F. Newborn is capable of digesting simple carbohydrates and protein but has difficulty with fats in formulas.
G. Immature cardiac (esophageal) sphincter may allow reflux of food when burped; may elevate crib after feeding.
H. Stomach capacity varies; approximately 15–30 ml.
I. First stool is meconium (black, tarry residue from lower intestine); usually passed within 12–24 hours after birth.
J. Transitional stools are thin and brownish green in color; after 3 days, milk stools are usually passed—loose and golden yellow for the breastfed infant, formed and pale yellow for the formula-fed infant. Stools may vary in number from 1 every feeding to 1–2/day.
K. Feeding patterns vary; newborn may nurse vigorously immediately after birth, or may need as long as several days to learn to suck effectively. Provide support and encouragement to new mothers during this time as infant feeding is a very emotional area for new mothers.

Hepatic

A. Liver responsible for changing hemoglobin (from breakdown of RBC) into unconjugated bilirubin, which is further changed into conjugated (water-soluble) bilirubin that can be excreted.
B. Excess unconjugated bilirubin can permeate the sclera and the skin, giving a jaundiced or yellow appearance to these tissues.
C. The liver of a mature infant can maintain the level of unconjugated bilirubin at less than 12 mg/dl. Higher levels indicate a possible dysfunction and the need for intervention.
D. This physiologic jaundice is considered normal in early newborns. It begins to appear after 24 hours, usually between 48–72 hours.

Temperature

A. Heat production in newborn accomplished by
  1. Metabolism of "brown fat," a special structure in newborn that is source of heat.
  2. Increased metabolic rate and activity.
B. Newborn cannot shiver as an adult does to release heat.
C. Newborn's body temperature drops quickly after birth; cold stress occurs easily.
D. Body stabilizes temperature in 8-10 hours if unstressed.
E. Cold stress increases oxygen consumption; may lead to metabolic acidosis and respiratory distress.

Immunologic

A. Newborn has passive acquired immunity from IgG from mother during pregnancy and passage of additional antibodies in colostrum and breast milk.
B. Newborn develops own antibodies during first 3 months, but is at risk for infection during first 6 weeks.
C. Ability to develop antibodies develops sequentially.

Neurologic/Sensory

Six States of Consciousness

A. Deep sleep
B. Light sleep: some body movements
C. Drowsy: occasional startle; eyes glazed
D. Quiet alert: few movements, but eyes open and bright
E. Active alert: active, occasionally fussy with much facial movement
F. Crying: much activity, eyes open or closed

Periods of Reactivity

A. First (birth through first 1-2 hours): newborn alert with good sucking reflex, irregular R/HR.
B. Second (4-8 hours after birth): may regurgitate mucus, pass meconium, and suck well
C. Equilibrium usually achieved by 8 hours of age.

Sleep Cycle

Newborn sleeps an average of 17 hours/day.

Hunger Cycle

Varies, depending on mode of feeding.
A. Breastfed infant may nurse every 2-3 hours.
B. Bottle-fed infant may be fed every 3-4 hours.

Special Senses

A. Sight: eyes are sensitive to light; newborn will fix and gaze at objects, especially those with black and white, regular patterns, but eye movements are uncoordinated.

B. Hearing: can hear before birth (24 weeks); newborn seems best attuned to human speech and its cadences.

C. Taste: sense of taste established; prefers sweet-tasting fluids; derives satisfaction as well as nourishment from sucking.

D. Smell: sense is developed at birth; newborn can identify own mother's breast milk by odor.

E. Touch: newborn is well prepared to receive tactile messages; mother demonstrates touch progression in initial bonding activities.

■ ASSESSMENT

Physical Examination

A. Weight
   1. Average between 2750 and 3629 g (6-8 lb) at term
   2. Initial loss of 5-8% of body weight normal during first few days; should be regained in 1-2 weeks

B. Length: average 45.7-55.9 cm (18-22 in)

C. Head circumference: average 33-35.5 cm (13-14 in); remeasure after several days if significant molding or caput succedaneum present

D. Chest circumference: average 1.9 cm ($^3/_4$ in) less than head

E. Abdominal girth may be measured if indicated. Consistent placement of tape is important for comparison, identification of abnormalities. Measurement is best done before feeding, as abdomen relaxes after a feeding.

F. Skin
   1. Color in Caucasian infants usually pink; varies with other ethnic backgrounds.
   2. Pigmentation increases after birth.
   3. Skin may be dry.
   4. Acrocyanosis of hands and feet normal for 24 hours; may develop "newborn rash" (erythema toxicum neonatorum).
   5. Small amounts of lanugo and vernix caseosa still seen.

G. Fontanels
   1. Anterior: diamond shaped
   2. Posterior: triangular
   3. Should be flat and open

H. Ears
   1. Should be even with canthi of eyes.
   2. Cartilage should be present and firm.

I. Eyes
   1. May be irritated by medication instillation, some edema/discharge present.
   2. Color is slate blue.
J. Nodule of tissue present in breasts.
K. Female genitalia
   1. Vernix seen between labia.
   2. Blood-tinged mucoid vaginal discharge (pseudomenstruation) from high levels of circulating maternal hormones.
L. Male genitalia
   1. Testes descended or in inguinal canal
   2. Rugae cover scrotum
   3. Meatus at tip of penis
M. Legs
   1. Bowed
   2. No click or displacement of head of femur observed when hips flexed and abducted
N. Feet
   1. Flat
   2. Soles covered with creases in fully mature infant
O. Muscle tone
   1. Predominantly flexed
   2. Occasional transient tremors of mouth and chin
   3. Newborn can turn head from side to side in prone position
   4. Needs head supported when held erect or lifted
P. Reflexes present at birth
   1. Rooting, sucking, and swallowing.
   2. Tonic neck, "fencing" attitude.
   3. Grasp: newborn's fingers curl around anything placed in palm.
   4. *Moro reflex*: symmetric and bilateral abduction and extension of arms and hands; thumb and forefinger form a C; the "embrace" reflex.
   5. *Startle reflex*: similar to Moro, but with hands clenched.
   6. *Babinski's sign*: flare of toes when foot stroked from base of heel along lateral edge to great toe.
Q. Cry
   1. Loud and vigorous.
   2. Heard when infant is hungry, disturbed, or uncomfortable.

Apgar Scoring

A. Used to evaluate the newborn in five specific categories at 1 and 5 minutes after birth.
B. The 1-minute score reflects transitional values.
C. The composite score at 5 minutes provides the best direction for the planning of newborn care.

D. Composite score interpretations
   1. 0-4: prognosis for newborn is grave.
   2. 5-7: infant needs specialized, intensive care.
   3. 7 or above: infant should do well in normal newborn nursery.

Gestational Age Assessment

After birth, direct examination of the infant leads to an accurate assessment of maturity. This is important, as complications may vary with maturity level: pre- and postmature infants, in general, have greater difficulty adapting to extra-uterine life.

A. Physical examination
   1. Skin: thickens with gestational age; may be dry/peeling if postmature.
   2. Lanugo: disappears as pregnancy progresses.
   3. Sole (plantar) creases: increase with gestational age (both depth and number).
   4. Areola of breast: at term, 5-10 mm in diameter.
   5. Ear: cartilage stiffens, recoil increases, and curvature of pinna increases with advancing gestational age.
   6. Genitalia: in the male, check for descended testicles and scrotal rugae; in the female, look for the labia majora to cover the labia minora and clitoris.

B. Neuromuscular assessment (best done after 24 hours)
   1. Resting posture: relaxed posture (extension) seen in the premature; flexion increases with maturity.
   2. Square window angle: flex hand onto underside of forearm, identify angle at which you feel resistance. Angle decreases with increasing gestational age.
   3. Arm recoil: flex infant's arms, extend for 5 seconds, then release. Note angle formed as arms recoil. Decreases with increasing gestational age.
   4. Popliteal angle: place infant on back, extend one leg, and measure angle at point of resistance. Angle becomes more acute as gestation progresses.
   5. Scarf sign: draw one arm across chest until resistance is felt; note relation of elbow to midline of chest. Resistance increases with advancing gestational age.
   6. Heel to ear: attempt to raise foot to ear, noting point at which foot slips from your grasp. Resistance increases with gestational age.

In performing gestational age assessments, the use of a specific form usually facilitates the ease and accuracy of the process.

■ ANALYSIS

Nursing diagnoses for the normal newborn are related to the potential for dysfunction in transition period and first few days of life.

DELEGATION TIP

The initial neonatal assessment is completed by the RN. Subsequent monitoring may be performed by ancillary staff. Bathing, feeding, and transferring the baby from the nursery may be performed by ancillary personnel.

■ PLANNING AND IMPLEMENTATION

Goals

A. Newborn will adapt to extrauterine life.
  1. Body temperature will be maintained.
  2. Normal breathing and adequate oxygenation will be established.
  3. Cardiovascular function will be stable.
  4. Nutrition and promotion of growth will be established.
B. Positive parent-infant relationship will be established.
C. Potential dysfunctions will be identified early.
D. Needed interventions will be implemented early.

Interventions

Delivery Room

A. Perform Apgar scoring at 1 and 5 minutes after birth.
B. Perform rapid, overall physical and neurologic exam.
  1. Identify obvious congenital anomalies.
  2. Count vessels in cord.
  3. Identify injuries from birth trauma.
C. Prevent heat loss.
  1. Dry infant immediately after birth.
  2. Wrap newborn warmly, cover head, or place in specially warmed area.
  3. Place newborn on warm surfaces (mother's body) or cover cool surfaces (e.g., scale).
  4. Minimize placement of newborn near cooler areas (windows, outside walls).
D. Maintain established respirations and heartbeat.
E. Identify mother and infant with matching bands.
F. Perform cord clamping if physician has not done so.
G. Allow parents to hold infant, or place in warmed unit.
H. Suction gently prn with bulb syringe.
 I. Administer oxygen prn.
 J. Promote bonding through early nursing if mother so desires, or by having parents hold newborn.

NURSING ALERT

Formula may be warmed to room temperature; do not microwave. Limiting time at each breast will not prevent sore nipples. Sore nipples are caued by incorrect positioning.

NURSING ALERT

Meconium stool that contains bile, epithelial cells, and amniotic cells is expected in 24 hours after birth in 90 % of newborns.

Nursery

A. Continue actions to prevent heat loss (temperature done rectally on admission then axillary, tympanic not accurate on infants).
B. When temperature stabilizes, perform complete physical and neurologic exam.
C. Administer medications as ordered.
  1. To prevent ophthalmia neonatorum, administration of 0.5% erythromycin or 1% tetracycline into conjunctival sac(s).
  2. Vitamin K: prophylactic dose to prevent hemorrhage.
  3. Hepatitis B vaccine in first 12 hours.
D. Measure and weigh newborn.
E. After temperature has stabilized, bathe and dress newborn, place in open crib.
F. Institute daily care routine.
  1. Take weight.
  2. Monitor temperature, apical pulse, respirations at least every shift.
  3. Suction prn.
  4. Bathe daily if ordered.
  5. Give diaper area care after each change.
  6. Continue assessment for anomalies.
  7. Allow umbilical cord to air dry by folding diaper below cord. Some institutions still use alcohol wipes.
  8. Institute feeding schedule as ordered.
  9. Note voidings and stools on daily basis.
G. Assess for physiologic jaundice.
  1. First manifests in the head area (test by depressing skin over bridge of nose) then progresses to chest (depress skin over sternum).

CLIENT TEACHING CHECKLIST

Instruction regarding neonatal care for the parents and significant others should include the following topics:

- cord care: fold diapers below cord, give sponge baths (include demonstration and return demonstration)
- circumcision care: clean penis, avoid baths until healing occurs
- voiding and elimination patterns: apply ointment to avoid contact with urine and feces
- feeding and preparing formula

2. Early feedings promote excretion of bilirubin in stool, diminishing incidence of jaundice.
3. Prevention of cold stress in newborn diminishes incidence of jaundice.
4. Loose, greenish stools and green-tinged urine are normal for these infants; advise mother.
5. These infants need extra fluids to prevent dehydration and replace fluids being excreted.
6. Advise parents that breast-fed infants may have increased jaundice.
   a. May not feed frequently enough in first 2 days and become dehydrated
   b. Breastmilk jaundice not a confirmed problem, usually an underfed baby.
H. Provide phototherapy if ordered, not usually required in physiologic jaundice unless levels rise rapidly or reach the high teens.
I. Monitor for pathologic jaundice.
   1. Appears at birth or in the first 24 hours.
   2. Bilirubin levels over 12 mg/dl.
J. Male infants may need circumcision care.
   1. Observe for bleeding.
   2. Note first voiding after circumcision.
   3. Clean area appropriately.
   4. Vaseline to penis to prevent sticking to diaper.
K. Perform screening tests before discharge (PKU, hypothyroidism, galactasemia, etc.).
L. Provide teaching and demonstrations as indicated for parents (e.g., feeding, burping, holding, diapering, bathing, positioning, safety).

■ EVALUATION

A. Newborn progress continually observed, normal vital signs for newborn maintained

B. No dysfunctional patterns discerned
C. No congenital anomalies identified
D. Parents comfortable with infant, have initiated bonding
E. Parents comfortable with newborn care
F. All necessary tests carried out at correct time
G. Evidence for continued growth and development at home is positive

■ VARIATIONS FROM NORMAL NEWBORN ASSESSMENT FINDINGS

Some variations from the normal assessment findings in the newborn are not indicative of any disorders; others, however, provide information about likely gestational age or the possibility of the existence of a more serious disorder.

Weight

A. Under 2500 g (5½ lb): small for gestational age (SGA)
B. Over 4100 g (9 lb): large for gestational age (LGA)

Length

A. Under 45.7 cm (18 in): SGA
B. Over 55.9 cm (22 in): LGA

Head Circumference

A. Under 31.7 cm (12½ in): microcephaly/SGA
B. Over 36.8 cm (14½ in): hydrocephaly/LGA

Blood Pressure

A. Variation with activity: normal
B. Major difference between upper and lower extremities: possible aortic coarctation

Pulse

A. Persistently under 120: possible heart block
B. Persistently over 170: possible respiratory distress syndrome

Temperature

A. Elevated: possible dehydration or infection
B. Temperature falls with low environmental temperature, late in cold stress, sepsis, cardiac disease.

Respirations

A. Under 25/minute: possibly result of maternal analgesia
B. Over 60/minute: possible respiratory distress

Skin

A. Milia (blocked sebaceous glands, usually on nose and chin) are essentially normal.
B. "Stork bites"
  1. Capillary hemangiomas above eyebrows and at base of neck under hairline are essentially normal.
  2. Raised capillary hemangiomas on areas other than face or neck are *not* normal findings.
C. Newborn rash (erythema toxicum neonatorum) is normal.
D. Mongolian spots (darkened areas of pigmentation over sacral area and buttocks) are normal and fade in early childhood. (Seen in Asian and African-American babies.)
E. Fingernail scratches are normal.
F. Excess lanugo: possible prematurity.
G. Vernix
  1. Decreases after 38 weeks, full-term usually has only in creases
  2. Excess: prematurity

Head

A. Fontanels
  1. Depressed: dehydration
  2. Bulging: increased intracranial pressure
B. Hair: coarse or brittle, possible endocrine disorder
C. Scalp: edema present at birth (*caput succedaneum*) from pressure of cervix against presenting part; crosses suture lines; disappears in 3–4 days without intervention.
D. Skull: collection of blood between a skull bone and its periosteum (*cephalhematoma*) from pressure during delivery; does not cross suture line; appears 12–24 hours after delivery; regresses in 3–6 weeks.
E. Eyes
  1. Edema from medications not uncommon
  2. Strabismus (occasional crossing of eyes) is normal
  3. Wide space between eyes is seen in fetal alcohol syndrome
F. Ears
  1. Lack of cartilage: possible prematurity
  2. Low placement: possible kidney disorder or Down's syndrome
G. Nose: copious drainage associated with syphilis
H. Mouth
  1. Thrush: appears as white patches in mouth; candida infection passed from mother during passage through birth canal.
  2. Tongue movement and excess salivation: possible esophageal atresia

Neck
Webbing; masses in muscle

Chest
Breast enlargement and milky secretion from breasts (witch's milk) is result of maternal hormones; self-limiting.

Cord
Fewer than three vessels may indicate congenital anomalies.

Female Genitalia
Pseudomenstruation is normal.

Male Genitalia
Misplaced urinary meatus
A. *Epispadias*: on upper surface of penis
B. *Hypospadias*: on under surface of penis

Upper Extremities
A. Extra fingers
B. Webbed fingers
C. Asymmetric movement: possible trauma or fracture

Lower Extremities
A. Extra toes
B. Webbed toes
C. Congenital hip dysplasia
D. Few creases on soles of feet: prematurity

Spine
Tuft of hair: possible occult spina bifida; assess pilonidal area for fistula.

Anus
Lack of meconium after 24 hours may indicate obstruction, disease.

REVIEW QUESTIONS

1. Which nursing action should be included in the care of the infant with a caput succedaneum?
   1. Aspiration of the trapped blood under the periosteum.
   2. Explanation to the parents about the cause/prognosis.
   3. Gentle rubbing in a circular motion to decrease size.
   4. Application of cold to reduce size.

2. A baby girl was born at 9:15 A.M. At 9:20 A.M. her heart rate was 132 beats/minute, she was crying vigorously, moving all extremities, and only her hands and feet were still slightly blue. The nurse should enter her Apgar score as
   1. 7.
   2. 8.
   3. 9.
   4. 10.

3. Which of the following findings in a newborn baby girl is normal?
   1. Passage of meconium within the first 24 hours.
   2. Respiratory rate of 70/minute at rest.
   3. Yellow skin tones at 12 hours of age.
   4. Bleeding from umbilicus.

4. The nursery nurse carries a newborn baby into his mother's room. The mother states, "I think my baby's afraid of me. Every time I make a loud noise, he jumps." The nurse should
   1. encourage her not to be so nervous with her baby.
   2. reassure her that this is a normal reflexive reaction for her baby.
   3. take the baby back to the nursery for a neurologic evaluation.
   4. wrap the baby more tightly in warm blankets.

5. A new mother asks how much weight her newborn will lose. The nurse replies
   1. none.
   2. 5%.
   3. 5–8%.
   4. 10–15%.

6. Which of the following findings in a 3-hour-old, full-term newborn would the nurse record as abnormal when assessing the head?

1. Two "soft spots" between the cranial bones.
2. Asymmetry of the head with overriding bones.
3. Head circumference 32 cm, chest 34 cm.
4. A sharply outlined, spongy area of edema.

7. The nurse collects the following data while assessing the skin of a 6-hour-old newborn: color pink with bluish hands and feet, some pale yellow papules with red base over trunk, small white spots on the nose, and a red area at the nape of the neck. The nurse's next action would be to

1. document findings as within normal range.
2. isolate infant pending diagnosis.
3. request a dermatology consultation.
4. document as indicators of malnutrition.

8. While performing the discharge assessment on a 2-day-old newborn, the nurse finds that after blanching the skin on the forehead, the color turns yellow. The nurse knows that this indicates

1. a normal biologic response.
2. an infectious liver condition.
3. an Rh incompatibility problem.
4. jaundice related to breast feeding.

9. A newborn is 2 days old and is being breastfed. The nurse finds that yesterday her stool was thick and tarry, today it's thinner and greenish brown; she voided twice since birth with some pink stains noted on the diaper. The nurse knows that these findings indicate

1. marked dehydration.
2. inadequate initial nutrition.
3. normal newborn elimination.
4. a need for medical consultation.

10. The nurse notes the following behaviors in a 6-hour-old, full-term newborn: occasional tremors of extremities, straightens arms and hands outward and flexes knees when disturbed, toes fan out when heel is stroked, and tries to walk when held upright. The nurse knows that these findings indicate

1. signs of drug withdrawal.
2. abnormal uncoordinated movements.
3. asymmetric muscle tone.
4. expected neurologic development.

11. While assessing a newborn, the nurse notes that the areola is flat with less than 0.5 cm of breast tissue. This finding indicates
    1. that infant is male.
    2. maternal hormonal depletion.
    3. intrauterine growth retardation.
    4. preterm gestational age.

12. The nurse's initial care plan for a full-term newborn includes the nursing diagnosis "risk of fluid volume depletion related to absence of intestinal flora." A related nursing intervention would be to
    1. administer glucose water or put to breast.
    2. assess first void and passing of meconium.
    3. administer vitamin K injection.
    4. send cord blood to lab for Coombs' test.

13. In the time immediately following birth, the nurse may delay instillation of eye medication primarily to
    1. check prenatal record to determine if prophylactic treatment is needed.
    2. ensure that initial eye saline irrigation is completed.
    3. enable mother to breast feed the infant in the first hour of life.
    4. facilitate eye contact and bonding between parents and newborn.

14. The nurses should include which of the following instructions in the care plan for a new mother who is breastfeeding her full-term newborn?
    1. Put to breast when infant shows readiness to feed.
    2. Breastfeed infant every 3 to 4 hours until discharge.
    3. Offer water feedings between breastfeedings.
    4. Feed infant when he shows hunger by crying.

15. In the delivery area, after ensuring that the newborn has established respirations, the next priority of the nurse should be to
    1. perform the Apgar score.
    2. place plastic clamp on cord.
    3. dry infant and provide warmth.
    4. ensure correct identification.

16. During the bath demonstration, a woman asks the nurse if it is OK to use baby powder because warm weather is coming. The nurse should respond
    1. "Just dust in on the diaper area only."
    2. "It's best not to use powder on infants."

3. "First use baby oil, then the powder."

4. "If the baby is just in a diaper he'll be cool."

17. Which of the following muscles would the nurse choose as the preferred site for a newborn's vitamin K injection?

    1. Gluteus medius.

    2. Mid-deltoid.

    3. Vastus lateralis.

    4. Rectus femoris.

18. The nurse knows that a mother understands proper cord care for her newborn when the client

    1. views a videotape on newborn hygiene care.

    2. reads a booklet on care of the newborn's cord stump.

    3. says she will apply Bacitracin ointment three times per day.

    4. cleans the cord and surrounding skin with an alcohol pad.

19. The nurse knows that more instruction on care of the circumcised infant is needed when the mother states,

    1. "I know to gently retract the foreskin after the area is healed."

    2. "At each diaper change I will squeeze water over the penis and pat dry."

    3. "I know not to disturb the yellow exudate that will form."

    4. "For the first day or so I'll apply a little A&D ointment."

20. The nurse knows that a new mother has a basic understanding of bottle feeding her infant when the client states,

    1. "I know not to prop the bottle until my baby is older."

    2. "With these little bottles, he should be able to finish them."

    3. "When I hold the bottle upside down, drops of milk should fall."

    4. "I should burp the baby about every 5-10 minutes."

ANSWERS AND RATIONALES

1. 2. Caput succedaneum (scalp edema) will regress in a few days without interventions and without residual damage.

2. 3. Acrocyanosis, where hands and feet are still slightly blue for the first 24 hours, is a normal variant in the newborn, but it rates a 1 on the Apgar scale. All the other descriptors are rated 2 on the Apgar scale, giving this newborn a total of 9.

3. 1. Meconium is usually passed during the first 24 hours of life.

4. 2. The startle reflex, normally present in neonates, is characterized by symmetric extension and abduction of the arms with fingers extended. The parent perceives this response as jumping.

5. 3. Within 3–4 days of birth, a weight loss of 5–8% is normal.

6. 3. The circumference of the newborn's head should be approximately 2 cm greater than the circumference of the chest at birth and will remain in this proportion for the next few months. Any differences in head size may indicate microcephaly (abnormal smallness of head) or hydrocephalus (increased cerebrospinal fluid within the ventricles of the brain).

7. 1. These findings of acrocyanosis (bluish discoloration of the hands and feet), erythema toxicum (newborn rash), milia, and a nevus flammeus (port wine stain) are all within the normal range for a full-term newborn.

8. 1. Physiologic jaundice occurs after the first 24 hours of life and is caused by accelerated destruction of fetal red blood cells (RBCs), impaired conjugation of bilirubin, and increased bilirubin reabsorption from the intestinal tract; there is no pathologic basis.

9. 3. Normal term newborns pass meconium within 8–24 hours of life; meconium is formed in utero and is thick, tarry, black (or dark green) in appearance. Transitional stool is a thinner brown to green. Normal voiding is 2 to 6 times daily; there may be innocuous pink stains ("brick dust spots") on the diaper from urates.

10. 4. Tremors are common in the full-term newborn; when a newborn is startled s/he will exhibit the Moro reflex, that is, s/he will straighten arms and hands outward while the knees flex; in a newborn the Babinski reflex is displayed by a fanning and extension of the toes (in adults the toes flex); and when held upright with feet lightly touching a surface, the newborn will put one foot in front of the other and "walk."

11. 4. At term gestation, the breast bud tissue will measure between 0.5 and 1 cm (5–10 mm).

12. 3. The newborn is at a high risk for hemorrhage due to an absence of intestinal flora (bacteria). Vitamin K, needed for the formation of prothrombin and proconvertin for blood coagulation, is usually synthesized by these bacteria in the colon; however, they are absent in the newborn's sterile gut. This problem is prevented by the administration of vitamin K following birth.

13. 4. The initial parental-newborn attachment period can be enhanced if the care providers keep routine investigations to a minimum, delay instillation of ophthalmic antibiotic for 1 hour, keep the room dim, and provide privacy; eye prophylaxis medication can cause chemical conjunctivitis, which may interfere with the baby's ability to focus on the parents' faces.

14. 1. It is important for the new mother to learn and respond to her infant's early feeding cues. Early cues that indicate a newborn is interested in feeding include hand-to-hand or hand-passing-mouth motion, whimpering, sucking, and rooting.

15. 3. After birth, the first priority is to maintain respirations, the second priority is to provide and maintain warmth; the newborn's temperature may fall 2–3°C after birth due mainly to evaporative losses; this triggers cold-induced metabolic responses and heat production.

16. 2. Powders and oils are not recommended for the neonate's skin; oils may clog the pores, and the small particles of powders may be inhaled by the neonate.

17. 3. The middle third of the vastus lateralis muscle in the thigh is the preferred site for an intramuscular injection in the newborn.

18. 4. Before discharge, parents should demonstrate proper cleaning of the cord stump by wiping it with an alcohol pad; they should know to do this 2 to 3 times a day until the cord falls off in 7–14 days.

19. 1. A circumcision is the surgical removal of the prepuce or foreskin from the tip of the penis; any foreskin that remains should not be retracted.

20. 3. The nipple should have a hole big enough to allow milk to flow in drops when the bottle is inverted; too large an opening may cause regurgitation, too small an opening can exhaust and upset the infant.

7

The High-Risk Infant

■ OVERVIEW

High-risk infants are those whose incidence of illness or death is increased because of prematurity, dysmaturity, postmaturity, physical problems, or birth complications. They are frequently the result of a high-risk pregnancy.

■ ASSESSMENT

A. History of high-risk pregnancy or other factor possibly affecting fetal development
B. Apgar scores in the delivery room
C. Head-to-toe assessment of the infant
D. Determination of gestational age

■ ANALYSIS

A. Alteration in respiratory function
B. Imbalanced nutrition: less than body requirements
C. Risk for impaired skin integrity
D. Ineffective tissue perfusion
E. Risk for injury
F. Impaired gas exchange
G. Ineffective thermoregulation
H. For parents of high-risk infants
    1. Ineffective coping
    2. Deficient knowledge
    3. Anticipatory grieving
    4. Powerlessness
    5. Social isolation

■ PLANNING AND IMPLEMENTATION
Goals

A. Needs of infant for physical care will be met.

1. Oxygen: respiratory functioning will be maintained.
2. Humidity and warmth: temperature will be regulated and cold stress prevented.
3. Adequate nutrition will be provided.
4. Tender handling: newborn will receive proper skin care and positioning.

B. Infection or other complications will be prevented.
C. Normal growth and development will be promoted.
D. Needs of parents for closeness with infant will be met; attachment/bonding will be promoted.

Interventions

A. Constantly monitor infant for subtle changes in condition and intervene promptly when necessary.
B. Conserve infant's energy and decrease physiologic stress.
C. Provide appropriate stimulation for infant growth and development.
D. Allow parents to express their reactions and feelings and assist them in attachment behaviors.
E. Teach parents care of infant in preparation for discharge.

■ EVALUATION

A. Infant's physical condition stabilized and improved on a steady basis
B. Infant's growth and development steady and appropriate
C. Parents demonstrated acceptance of and comfort with infant's condition
D. Parents demonstrated comfort and confidence with infant care at discharge

■ HIGH-RISK DISORDERS

The Premature Infant

A. General information
   1. Any infant born before the end of the 37th week of pregnancy
   2. Weight usually less than 2500 g (5½ lb)
   3. Causes include
      a. Maternal factors: age, smoking, poor nutrition, placental problems, preeclampsia/eclampsia
      b. Fetal factors: multiple pregnancy, infection, intrauterine growth retardation (IUGR)
      c. Other: socioeconomic status, environmental exposure to harmful substance
   4. Severity of problems related to level of maturity: the earlier the infant is born, the greater the chance of complications.
   5. Major complicating conditions
      a. Respiratory distress syndrome
      b. Thermoregulatory problems
      c. Conservation of energy

      d. Infection

      e. Hemorrhage

B. Assessment findings

    1. Respiratory system

      a. Insufficient surfactant

      b. Apneic episodes

      c. Retractions, nasal flaring, grunting, seesaw pattern of breathing, cyanosis

      d. Increased respiratory rate

    2. Thermoregulation: body temperature fluctuates easily (premature newborn has less subcutaneous fat and muscle mass)

    3. Nutritional status

      a. Poor sucking and swallowing reflexes

      b. Poor gag and cough reflexes

    4. Skin: lack of subcutaneous fat; reddened; translucent

    5. Drainage from umbilicus/eyes

    6. Cardiovascular

      a. Petechiae caused by fragile capillaries and prolonged prothrombin time

      b. Increased bleeding at injection sites

    7. Neuromuscular

      a. Poor muscle tone

      b. Weak reflexes

      c. Weak, feeble cry

C. Nursing interventions

    1. Maintain respirations at less than 60/minute, check every 1-2 hours.

    2. Administer oxygen as ordered; check concentration every 2 hours to avoid retrolental fibroplasia while providing adequate oxygenation.

    3. Auscultate breath sounds to assess lung expansion.

    4. Encourage breathing with gentle rubbing of back and feet.

    5. Suction as needed.

    6. Reposition every 1-2 hours for maximum lung expansion and prevention of exhaustion.

    7. Monitor blood gases and electrolytes.

    8. Maintain thermoneutral body temperature; prevent cold stress.

    9. Maintain appropriate humidity level.

   10. Monitor for signs of infection; these infants have little antibody production and decreased resistance.

   11. Feed according to abilities.

   12. Monitor sucking reflex; if poor, gavage feeding indicated. Most preterm infants require at least some gavage feeding as it diminishes the effort required for sucking while improving the caloric intake.

   13. Use "preemie" nipple if bottle-feeding.

   14. Monitor I&O, weight gain or loss; these infants are easily dehydrated, with poor electrolyte balance.

NURSING ALERT

Pulse oximeter readings of 88–92% reflect a safe clinical range. Readings above or below this range require intervention.

NURSING ALERT

The heel is the preferred site to test blood glucose; warm the foot prior to obtaining blood sample to increase circulation.

15. Monitor for hypoglycemia and hyperbilirubinemia.
16. Handle carefully; organize care to minimize disturbances.
17. Provide skin care with special attention to cleanliness and careful positioning to prevent breakdown.
18. Monitor heart rate and pattern at least every 1–2 hours; listen apically for 1 full minute.
19. Monitor potential bleeding sites (umbilicus, injection sites, skin); these infants have lowered clotting factors.
20. Monitor overall growth and development of infant; check weight, length, head circumference.
21. Provide tactile stimulation when caring for or feeding infant.
22. Provide complete explanations for parents.
23. Encourage parental involvement in infant's care.
24. Provide support for parents; refer to self-help group or other parents if necessary.
25. Promote parental confidence with infant care before discharge.

The Dysmature Infant (SGA)

A. General information
   1. Birth weight in the lowest 10th percentile at term
   2. Causes: discounting heredity, possibly intrauterine growth retardation, infections, malformations
B. Assessment findings
   1. Skin: loose and dry, little fat, little muscle mass
   2. Small body makes skull look larger than normal
   3. Sunken abdomen
   4. Thin, dry umbilical cord
   5. Little scalp hair
   6. Wide skull sutures
   7. Respiratory distress; may have had hypoxic episodes in utero

       8. Hypoglycemia

       9. Tremors

     10. Weak cry

     11. Lethargic

     12. Cool to touch

C. Nursing interventions

    1. Care of SGA infant is similar in many instances to care of preterm infant.

    2. Tailor high-level nursing care to meet specific needs of infant with regard to functioning of all body systems, psychologic growth and development, parental support and teaching, and prevention of complications.

The Postmature Infant

A. General information

    1. Born after the completion of 42 weeks of pregnancy

    2. Problems caused by progressively less efficient actions of placenta

B. Assessment findings

    1. Skin

       a. Vernix and lanugo completely disappeared

       b. Dry, cracked, parchmentlike appearance of skin

       c. Color: yellow to green from meconium staining

    2. Depleted subcutaneous fat; old looking

    3. Hard nails extending beyond fingertips

    4. Signs of birth injury or poor tolerance of birth process

C. Nursing interventions

    1. Nursing care of the postmature infant has many characteristics in common with the care given to the premature infant.

    2. Design high-level nursing care to identify the infant's specific physical and psychologic needs; monitor functioning of all body systems, growth and development, parental support and teaching, and prevention of complications.

■ SPECIAL CONDITIONS IN THE NEONATE

Hyperbilirubinemia

A. General information

    1. Elevated serum level of bilirubin in the newborn results in jaundice or yellow color of body tissues.

    2. In physiologic jaundice, average increase from 2 mg/dl in cord blood to 6 mg/dl by 72 hours; not exceeding 12 mg/dl.

    3. Level at which a newborn will sustain damage to body cells (especially brain cells) from high concentrations of bilirubin is termed pathologic.

CLIENT TEACHING CHECKLIST

Teach the parents to:

- Feed the infant every 2–3 hours to prevent dehydration.
- Observe for dry mucous membranes.
- Keep the baby warm; major heat loss occurs through the head.

4. May result from immaturity of liver, Rh or ABO incompatibility, infection, birth trauma with subsequent bleeding (cephalhematoma), maternal diabetes, hypothermia, medications.
5. Major complication is *kernicterus* (brain damage caused by high levels of unconjugated bilirubin).

B. Assessment findings
1. Pathologic jaundice usually appears early, up to 24 hours after birth; represents a process ongoing before birth
2. Usual pattern of progression is from head to feet. Blanch skin over bony area or look at conjunctiva and buccal membranes in dark-skinned infants
3. Pallor
4. Dark, concentrated urine (often dehydrated)
5. Behavior changes (irritability, lethargy)
6. Polycythemia
7. Increased serum bilirubin (direct, indirect, and total)

C. Nursing interventions
1. Identify conditions predisposing to hyperbilirubinemia, especially positive coombs test (test on cord blood for presence of maternal antibodies).
2. Prevent progression or complications of jaundice.
3. Assess jaundice levels (visually, lab tests) as needed.
4. Prevent conditions that contribute to development of hyperbilirubinemia (e.g., cold stress, hypoxia, acidosis, hypoglycemia, dehydration, infection).
5. Provide adequate hydration.
6. Implement phototherapy if ordered; use of blue lights overhead, blanket-device wrapped around infant (Wallaby), or bili-bed.
   a. Overhead unit
      1) Unclothe infant for maximum skin exposure; minimal diaper
      2) Cover eyes to prevent retinal damage
      3) Carefully monitor temperature
      4) Monitor temperature carefully
      5) Remove baby from warmer and uncover eyes for feedings
      6) Ensure feedings every 3 hours

   b. Wallaby blanket
      1) Baby at bedside—explain care of unit to mother
      2) Keep unit on for feedings, eyes remain uncovered
      3) Other care as above
   7. Explain all tests and procedures to parents.
   8. Support parents with information on procedures.

Hemolytic Disease of the Newborn (Erythroblastosis Fetalis)

A. General information
   1. Characterized by RBC destruction in the newborn, with resultant anemia and hyperbilirubinemia
   2. Possibly caused by Rh or ABO incompatibility between the mother and the fetus (antigen/antibody reaction)
   3. Mechanisms of Rh incompatibility
      a. Sensitization of Rh-negative woman by transfusion of Rh-positive blood
      b. Sensitization of Rh-negative woman by presence of Rh-positive RBCs from her fetus conceived with Rh-positive man
      c. Approximately 65% of infants conceived by this combination of parents will be Rh positive.
      d. Mother is sensitized by passage of fetal Rh-positive RBCs through placenta, either during pregnancy (break/leak in membrane) or at the time of separation of the placenta after delivery.
      e. This stimulates the mother's immune response system to produce anti-Rh-positive antibodies that attack fetal RBCs and cause hemolysis.
      f. If this sensitization occurs during pregnancy, the fetus is affected in utero; if sensitization occurs at the time of delivery, subsequent pregnancies may be affected.
   4. ABO incompatibility
      a. Same underlying mechanism
      b. Mother is blood type O; infant is A, B, or AB.
      c. Reaction in ABO incompatibility is less severe.
B. Rh incompatibility
   1. First pregnancy: mother may become sensitized, baby rarely affected
   2. Indirect Coombs' test (tests for anti-Rh-positive antibodies in mother's circulation) performed during pregnancy at first visit and again about 28 weeks' gestation. If indirect Coombs' test is negative at 28 weeks, a small dose (MicRho gam) is given prophylactically to prevent sensitization in the third trimester. RhoGam may also be given after second trimester amniocentesis.
   3. If positive, levels are titrated to determine extent of maternal sensitization and potential effect on fetus.

4. Direct Coombs' test done on cord blood at delivery to determine presence of anti-Rh-positive antibodies on fetal RBCs.
5. If both indirect and direct Coombs' tests are negative (no formation of anti-Rh-positive antibodies) and infant is Rh positive, then Rh-negative mother can be given RhoGam (Rho[D] human immune globulin) to prevent development of anti-Rh-positive antibodies as the result of sensitization from present (just-terminated) pregnancy.
6. In each pregnancy, an Rh-negative mother who carries an Rh-positive fetus can receive RhoGam to protect future pregnancies if the mother has had negative indirect Coombs' tests and the infant has had a negative direct Coombs' test.
7. If mother has been sensitized (produced anti-Rh-positive antibodies), RhoGam is not indicated.
8. RhoGam must be injected into unsensitized mother's system within first 24 hours if possible, by 72 hours at latest.

C. ABO incompatibility
1. Reaction less severe than with Rh incompatibility
2. Firstborn may be affected because type O mother may have anti-A and anti-B antibodies even before pregnancy.
3. Fetal RBCs with A, B, or AB antigens evoke less severe reaction on part of mother, thus fewer anti-A, anti-B, or anti-AB antibodies are produced.
4. Clinical manifestations of ABO incompatibility are milder and of shorter duration than those of Rh incompatibility.
5. Care must be taken to observe for hemolysis and jaundice.

D. Assessment findings
1. Jaundice and pallor within first 24–36 hours
2. Anemia
3. Erythropoiesis
4. Enlarged placenta
5. Edema and ascites

E. Nursing interventions
1. Determine blood type and Rh early in pregnancy.
2. Determine results of indirect Coombs' test early in pregnancy and again at 28–32 weeks.
3. Determine results of direct Coombs' test on cord blood (type and Rh, hemoglobin and hematocrit).
4. Administer RhoGam IM to mother as ordered.
5. Monitor carefully infants of Rh-negative and Type O mothers for jaundice.
6. Set up phototherapy as ordered by physician and monitor infant during therapy.
7. Instruct parents if home device will be used.
8. Support parents with explanations and information.

Neonatal Sepsis

A. General information
   1. Associated with the presence of pathogenic microorganisms in the blood, especially gram-negative organisms (*E. coli, Aerobacter, Proteus,* and *Klebsiella*), and gram-positive group B beta-hemolytic streptococci.
   2. Contributing factors
      a. Prolonged rupture of membranes (more than 24 hours)
      b. Prolonged or difficult labor
      c. Maternal infection
      d. Infection in hospital personnel
      e. Aspiration at birth or later
      f. Poor handwashing techniques among staff
B. Assessment findings
   1. Behavioral changes: lethargy, irritability, poor feeding
   2. Frequent periods of apnea
   3. Jaundice
   4. Hypothermia or low-grade fever
   5. Vomiting, diarrhea
C. Nursing interventions
   1. Perform cultures as indicated/ordered.
   2. Administer antibiotics for 3 days till 72 hour cultures back if negative, discontinue; if positive, continue with full course of specific antibiotics
   3. Prevent heat loss.
   4. Administer oxygen as indicated.
   5. Maintain hydration.
   6. Monitor vital signs (temperature, pulse, respirations) frequently.
   7. Weigh daily.
   8. Stroke back and feet gently to stimulate breathing if infant is apneic.
   9. Promote parental attachment and involvement in newborn care.

Hypoglycemia

A. General information
   1. Less-than-normal amount of glucose in the blood of the neonate
   2. Common in infants of diabetic mothers (IDM), especially type III: these infants usually LGA (macrosomic) due to high maternal glucose levels that have crossed placenta, stimulating the fetal pancreas to secrete more insulin, which then acts as growth hormone.
   3. At birth, with loss of supply of maternal glucose, newborn may become hypoglycemic.
   4. Large size may have caused traumatic vaginal birth, or may have necessitated cesarean birth.

5. Hypoglycemia can also occur in infants who are full term, SGA, postterm, septic, or with any condition that subjects the infant to stress.
B. Assessment findings
   1. May be born prematurely due to complications
   2. Although LGA, IDMs may be immature/dysmature
   3. Higher incidence of congenital anomalies in IDMs
   4. General appearance
      a. Puffy body
      b. Enlarged organs
   5. Tremors, feeding difficulty, irregular respirations, lethargy, hypothermia
   6. Hypocalcemia and hyperbilirubinemia
   7. Respiratory distress
   8. Blood glucose levels below 40 mg/dl (20 mg/dl in premature infant) using Dextristix
C. Nursing interventions
   1. Provide high-level nursing care similar to that for premature/dysmature infant.
   2. Assess blood glucose level at frequent intervals, beginning ½–1 hour after birth in at-risk infants.
   3. Feed hypoglycemic infant according to nursery protocol (formula or breast preferred) if suck/swallow reflex present and coordinated.
   4. Poor suck-swallow or lack of serum response to PO feeding, administer IV glucose.

Infant Born to Addicted Mother

A. General information
   1. Substance may be alcohol, heroin, morphine, or any other addictive drug.
   2. Mother usually seeks prenatal care only when labor begins and has frequently taken a dose of addictive substance before seeking help, delaying withdrawal symptoms 12–24 hours.
   3. Withdrawal symptoms in the neonate may be noticed within 24 hours.
B. Assessment findings
   1. Infants born to alcohol-abusing mothers may have facial anomalies, fine-motor dysfunction, genital abnormalities (especially females), and cardiac defects; may be SGA (also called the *fetal alcohol syndrome*)
   2. Hyperirritability and hyperactivity
   3. High-pitched cry common
   4. Respiratory distress, tachypnea, excessive secretions
   5. Vomiting and diarrhea
   6. Elevated temperature
   7. Other signs of withdrawal: sneezing; sweating; yawning; short, nonquiet sleep; frantic sucking

C. Nursing interventions
   1. Reduce external stimuli.
   2. Handle minimally.
   3. Swaddle infant and hold close when handling.
   4. Monitor infant's vital signs.
   5. Suction/resuscitate as required.
   6. Feed frequently, with small amounts.
   7. Measure I&O.
   8. Provide careful skin care.
   9. Administer medications if ordered (may use phenobarbital or paragoric).
   10. Involve parents in care if possible.
   11. Inform parents of infant's condition/progress.

Respiratory Distress Syndrome (RDS)

A. General information
   1. Symptoms found almost exclusively in the preterm infant.
   2. Deficiency of surfactant increases surface tension, which causes alveolar collapse.
   3. When women are likely to deliver prematurely, betamethasone is given IM in two doses, 12 hours apart.
   4. Additional factors: hypoxia, hypothermia, acidosis
   5. Sequelae of RDS may include
      a. Patent ductus arteriosus
      b. Hyperbilirubinemia
      c. Retrolental fibroplasia: retinal changes, visual impairment and eventually blindness, resulting from too-high oxygen levels during treatment
      d. Bronchopulmonary dysplasia (BPD): damage to the alveolar epithelium of the lungs related to high oxygen concentrations and positive pressure ventilation. May be difficult to wean infant from ventilator, but most recover and have normal X-rays at 6 months to 2 years.
      e. Necrotizing enterocolitis (below).
B. Assessment findings
   1. Respiratory rate of over 60/minute
   2. Retractions, grunting, cyanosis, nasal flaring, chin lag
   3. Increased apical pulse
   4. Hypothermia
   5. Decreased activity level
   6. Elevated levels of carbon dioxide
   7. Metabolic acidosis
   8. X-rays show atelectasis and density in alveoli.
C. Nursing interventions
   1. Maintain infant's body temperature at 97.6°F (36.2°C).

2. Provide sufficient caloric intake for size, age, and prevention of catabolism (usually IV glucose with gradual increase in feedings); nasogastric tube may be used.
3. Organize care for minimal handling of infant.
4. Administer oxygen therapy as ordered.
   a. Monitor oxygen concentration every 2–4 hours; maintain less than 40% concentration if possible.
   b. Oxygen may be administered by hood, nasal prongs, intubation, or mask.
   c. Oxygen may be at atmospheric or increased pressure.
   d. Continuous positive air pressure (CPAP) or positive end-expiratory pressure (PEEP) may be used.
   e. Oxygen should be warmed and humidified.
5. Monitor infant's blood gases.
6. If intubated, suction (for less than 5 seconds) prn using sterile catheter.
7. Auscultate breath sounds.
8. Provide chest physiotherapy, postural drainage, and percussion if ordered.
9. Encourage parental involvement in care (visiting, stroking infant, talking).
10. Administer surfactant via endotracheal tube and other medications as ordered.

Necrotizing Enterocolitis (NEC)

A. General information
   1. An ischemic attack to the intestine resulting in thrombosis and infarction of affected bowel, mucosal ulcerations, pseudomembrane formation, and inflammation.
   2. Bacterial action (*E. coli, Klebsiella*) complicates the process, producing sepsis.
   3. May be precipitated by any event in which blood is shunted away from the intestine to the heart and brain (e.g., fetal distress, low Apgar score, RDS, prematurity, neonatal shock, and asphyxia).
   4. Average age at onset is 4 days.
   5. Now that severely ill infants are surviving, NEC is encountered more frequently.
   6. May ultimately cause bowel perforation and death.
   7. Less common in breastfed premature infants.
B. Medical management
   1. Parenteral antibiotics
   2. Gastric decompression
   3. Correction of acidosis and fluid electrolyte imbalances
   4. Surgical removal of the diseased intestine

C. Assessment findings
   1. History indicating high-risk group
   2. Findings related to sepsis
      a. Temperature instability
      b. Apnea, labored respirations
      c. Cardiovascular collapse
      d. Lethargy or irritability
   3. Gastrointestinal symptoms
      a. Abdominal distension and tenderness
      b. Vomiting or increased gastric residual
      c. Poor feeding
      d. Hematest positive stools
      e. X-rays showing air in the bowel wall, adynamic ileus, and bowel wall thickening
D. Nursing interventions
   1. Carefully assess infants at risk for early recognition of symptoms.
   2. Discontinue oral feedings, insert nasogastric tube.
   3. Prevent trauma to abdomen by avoiding diapers and planning care for minimal handling.
   4. Maintain acid-base balance by administering fluids and electrolytes as ordered.
   5. Administer antibiotics as ordered.
   6. Stroke infant's hands and head and talk to infant as much as possible.
   7. Provide visual and auditory stimulation.
   8. Inform parents of progress and support them in expressing their fears and concerns.

Phenylketonuria (PKU)

A. General information
   1. Inability to metabolize phenylalanine to tyrosine because of an autosomal recessive inherited disorder causing an inborn error of metabolism
   2. Phenylalanine is a composite of almost all proteins: **the danger to the infant is immediate**.
   3. High levels of phenylketones affect brain cells, causing mental retardation.
   4. Initial screening for diagnosis of PKU is made via the Guthrie test, done after the infant has ingested protein for a minimum of 24 hours.
   5. Secondary screening
      a. Done when the infant is about 6 weeks old.
      b. Test fresh urine with a Phenistix, which changes color.
      c. Parents send in a prepared sheet marking the color.
   6. These tests, mandatory in many states, allow the early diagnosis of the disorder, and dietary interventions to minimize or prevent complications.

B. Assessment findings
   1. Phenylalanine levels greater than 8 mg/dl are diagnostic for PKU.
   2. Newborn appears normal; may be fair with decreased pigmentation.
   3. Untreated PKU can result in failure to thrive, vomiting, and eczema; by about 6 months, signs of brain involvement appear.
C. Nursing interventions
   1. Restrict protein intake.
   2. Substitute a low-phenylalanine formula (Lofenalac) for either mother's milk or formula.
   3. Provide special food lists for parents.

REVIEW QUESTIONS

1. In differentiating physiologic jaundice from pathologic jaundice, which of the following facts is most important?
   1. Mother is 37 years of age.
   2. Infant is a term newborn.
   3. Unconjugated bilirubin level is 6 mg/dl on third day.
   4. Appears at 12 hours after birth.

2. A newborn is receiving phototherapy. To meet safety needs while he is undergoing phototherapy, the nurse would
   1. limit fluid intake.
   2. cover the infant's eyes while he is under the light.
   3. keep him clothed to prevent skin burns.
   4. make sure the light is not closer than 24 inches.

3. The morning temperature on a newborn is 97.6°F (36.4°C). In order to prevent cold stress, which nursing action should be included in the plan of care? Teach the mother to
   1. keep the baby's head covered.
   2. keep the baby unwrapped.
   3. turn up the thermostat in the nursery.
   4. use warm water for the bath.

4. A diabetic woman has a problem-free prenatal course and delivers a full-term 9 lb 2 oz girl. At 1 hour after birth, the baby exhibits tremors. The nurse performs a heel stick and a Dextrostix test. The result is 40 mg/dl. The nurse concludes that these symptoms are most likely caused by

1. hypoglycemia.
2. hypokalemia.
3. hypothermia.
4. hypercalcemia.

5. A newborn weighs 1450 g, has weak muscle tone, with extremities in an extended position while at rest. The pinna is flat and does not readily recoil. Very little breast tissue is palpable. The soles have deep indentations over the upper one-third. Based on these data, what should the nurse know about the baby's gestational age?

   1. Full-term infant, 38–42 weeks' gestation.
   2. Premature infant, less than 24 weeks' gestation.
   3. Premature infant, 29–33 weeks' gestation.
   4. Postterm infant greater than 42 weeks' gestation.

6. A premature infant at 6 hours old, has respirations of 64, mild nasal flaring, and expiratory grunting. She is pink in room air, temperature is 36.5°C. The baby's mother ruptured membranes 36 hours prior to delivery. Which measures should the nurse include in the plan of care?

   1. Have respiratory therapy set up a respirator since respiratory failure is imminent. Get blood gases every hour.
   2. Encourage mother/infant interaction. Rooming in as soon as stable. Monitor vital signs every eight hours.
   3. Observe for signs of sepsis. Cultures if ordered. Monitor vital signs at least every 2 hours for the first 24 hours. Encourage family interaction with infant.
   4. Radiant warmer for first 48 hours. Vital signs every hour. Restrict visitation due to risk of infection.

7. During the assessment of a 2-day-old infant with bruising and a cephalhematoma, the nurse notes jaundice of the face and trunk. The baby is also being breastfed. Bilirubin level is 10 mg/dl. What is the most likely interpretation of these findings?

   1. Hyperbilirubinemia due to the bruising and cephalhematoma.
   2. Pathologic jaundice requiring exchange transfusion.
   3. Breast milk jaundice.
   4. Hyperbilirubinemia due to blood group incompatibility.

8. A 6-hour-old newborn has been diagnosed with erythroblastosis fetalis. The nurse understands that this condition is caused by

   1. ABO blood group incompatibility between the father and infant.
   2. Rh incompatibility between the mother and infant.

3. ABO blood group incompatibility between the mother and infant.

4. Rh incompatibility between father and infant.

9. An Rh negative mother has just given birth to an Rh positive infant. She had a negative indirect Coombs' test at 38 weeks' gestation and her infant had a negative direct Coombs' test. What should the nurse know about these tests?

   1. Although her infant is Rh positive, she has no antibodies to the Rh factor. RhoGam should be given.

   2. She has demonstrated antibodies to the Rh factor. She should not have any more children.

   3. She has formed antigens against the Rh factor. RhoGam must be given to the infant.

   4. Since her infant is Rh positive, the Coombs' tests are meaningless.

10. An infant was born at 38 weeks' gestation to a heroin-addicted mother. At birth, the baby had Apgar scores of 5 at 1 minute and 6 at 5 minutes. Birthweight was at the 10th percentile for gestational age. What should the nurse include in the baby's plan of care?

    1. Administer methadone to diminish symptoms of heroin withdrawal.

    2. Promote parent-infant attachment by encouraging rooming-in.

    3. Observe for signs of jaundice because this is a common complication.

    4. Place in a quiet area of the nursery and swaddle with hands near mouth to promote more organized behavioral state.

11. A 36-week-gestation infant had tachypnea, nasal flaring, and intercostal retractions that increased over the first 6 hours of life. The baby was treated with IV fluids and oxygen. Which of the following assessments suggests to the nurse that the baby is improving?

    1. The baby has see-saw respirations with coarse breath sounds.

    2. The baby's respiratory rate is 50 and pulse is 136, no nasal flaring is observed.

    3. The baby has a pH of 6.97 and pO_2 of 61 on 40% oxygen.

    4. The baby has gained 150 g in the 12 hours since birth.

12. You are caring for an infant. During your assessment you note a flattened philtrum, short palpebral fissures, and birth weight and head circumference below the fifth percentile for gestational age. The infant has a poor suck. Which of the following is the best interpretation of this data?

    1. Down syndrome.

    2. Fetal alcohol syndrome.

    3. Turner's syndrome.

    4. Congenital syphilis.

13. A 2-week-old premature infant with abdominal distention, significant gastric aspirate prior to feeding, and bloody stools has also had episodes of apnea and bradycardia and temperature instability. What should the nurse include in the plan of care for this infant?

    1. Increase feeding frequency to every 2 hours.

    2. Place the infant on seizure precautions.

    3. Place the infant in strict isolation to prevent infection of other infants.

    4. Monitor infant carefully including blood pressure readings and measurements of abdominal girth.

14. A mother is taking her newborn home from the hospital at 18 hours after birth. As the nurse is giving discharge instructions, which response best validates her understanding of PKU testing?

    1. "I know you stuck my baby's heel today for that PKU test and that my doctor will recheck the test when I bring her for her 1 month appointment."

    2. "After I start my baby on cereal, I will return for a follow-up blood test."

    3. "I will have a visiting nurse come to the house each day for the first week to check the PKU test."

    4. "I will bring my baby back to the hospital or doctor's office to have a repeat PKU no later than 1 week from today."

ANSWERS AND RATIONALES

1. Time is one of the most important criteria in differentiating physiologic from pathologic jaundice. Physiologic jaundice appears after 24 hours. When jaundice appears earlier, it may be pathologic.

2. The infant receiving phototherapy should have a covering put over his eyes to protect them from light.

3. The baby's head should be kept covered. The head is the greatest source of heat loss.

4. Tremors are symptoms of the neonatal hypoglycemia. The baby of a diabetic mother is at high risk for hypoglycemia because the infant's insulin levels are high before birth and continue high even though the infant has suddenly lost the influx of glucose. Immediate administration of IV glucose will be ordered for the infant.

5. A birth weight of 1450 g is the mean weight for an infant at 30 weeks' gestation, but falls within the 10–90th percentiles for infants between 29 and 33 weeks' gestation. The diminished muscle tone and extension of

extremities at rest are also characteristic of this gestational age. The sole creases described are actually most characteristic of an infant between 32 and 34 weeks' gestation.

6. Prolonged rupture of membranes places this premature infant at risk for sepsis. Frequent monitoring of vital signs, color, activity level, and overall behavior is particularly important because changes may provide early cues to a developing infection. Family interaction with the infant should always be a part of the nursing plan.

7. Although hyperbilirubinemia is common in newborns, certain factors increase the likelihood of early appearance of visible jaundice. Cold stress, bruising at delivery, cephalhematoma, asphyxiation, prematurity, breastfeeding, and poor feeding are all factors that may lead to hyperbilirubinemia in otherwise normal infants.

8. Erythroblastosis fetalis results when an Rh negative woman makes antibodies against her Rh positive fetus. The antibodies attack fetal red cells.

9. Since the indirect and direct Coombs' tests were negative, antibodies to Rh have not developed. She should have RhoGam to prevent antibody formation.

10. Neonatal withdrawal is a common occurrence in heroin addiction. Placing the baby in a quiet area and swaddling may promote state organization and minimize some symptoms. Medication may be needed to control hyperirritability.

11. The baby's respiratory rate and pulse are within normal limits and the nasal flaring is no longer present.

12. Although a medical diagnosis cannot be made from the assessment data, all of the findings noted are commonly seen in infants with fetal alcohol syndrome.

13. The infant's prematurity is the major risk factor for necrotizing enterocolitis, which affects 1–15% of all infants in NICU. Usual nonsurgical treatment includes antibiotic therapy, making the infant NPO, frequent monitoring, and respiratory and circulatory support as needed.

14. One additional PKU test within the first week of life will validate whether PKU disease is present. The infant should have been on breast milk or formula for 48 hours prior to the test.

8

Conditions of the Female Reproductive System

■ FERTILITY AND INFERTILITY

Infertility

General Information

CHAPTER OUTLINE

Fertility and Infertility

Menstrual Disorders

Infectious Disorders

A. Inability to conceive after at least 1 year of unprotected sexual relations
B. Inability to deliver a live infant after three consecutive pregnancies
C. For the male, inability to impregnate a female partner within the same conditions
D. May be primary (never been pregnant/never impregnated) or secondary (pregnant once, then unable to conceive or carry again)
E. Affects approximately 10-15% of all couples
F. Tests for infertility can include:
   1. For the female
      a. Examination of basal body temperature and cervical mucus and identification of time of ovulation
      b. Plasma progesterone level: assesses corpus luteum
      c. Hormone analysis: endocrine function
      d. Endometrial biopsy: receptivity of endometrium
      e. Postcoital test: sperm placement and cervical mucus
      f. Hysterosalpingography: tubal patency/uterine cavity
      g. Rubin's test: tubal patency (uses carbon dioxide)
      h. Pelvic ultrasound: visualization of pelvic tissues
      i. Laparoscopy: visual assessment of pelvic/abdominal organs; performance of minor surgeries
   2. For the male
      a. Sperm analysis: assesses composition, volume, motility, agglutination.
      b. There are fewer assessment tests as well as interventions and successes for male infertility.

149

Medical Management

A. Infertility of female partner, causes and therapy
   1. Congenital anomalies (absence of organs, improperly formed or abnormal organs): surgical treatment may help in some situations but cannot replace absent structures.
   2. Irregular/absent ovulation (ovum released irregularly or not at all): endocrine therapy with clomiphene citrate (Clomid)/menotropins (Pergonal) may induce ovulation; risk of ovarian hyperstimulation and release of multiple ova.
   3. Tubal factors (fallopian tubes blocked or scarred from infection, surgery, endometriosis, neoplasms): treatment may include antibiotic therapy, surgery, hysterosalpingogram.
   4. Uterine conditions (endometrium unreceptive, infected): removal of an IUD, antibiotic therapy, or surgery may be helpful.
   5. Vaginal/cervical factors (hostile mucus, sperm allergies, altered pH due to infection): treatment with antibiotics, proper vaginal hygiene, or artificial insemination may be utilized.
B. Infertility of male partner, causes and therapy
   1. Impotence: may be helped by psychologic counseling/penile implants, medication.
   2. Low/abnormal sperm count (fewer than 20 million/ml semen, low motility, more than 40% abnormal forms): there is no good therapy, use of hormone replacement therapy has had little success.
   3. Varicocele (varicosity within spermatic cord): ligation may be successful.
   4. Infection in any area of the male reproductive system (may affect ability to impregnate): appropriate antibiotic therapy is advised.
   5. Social habits (use of nicotine, alcohol, other drugs; clothes that keep scrotal sac too close to warmth of body): changing these habits may reverse low/absent fertility.
C. Alternatives for infertile couples include
   1. Artificial insemination by husband or donor
   2. In vitro fertilization
   3. Adoption
   4. Surrogate parenting
   5. Embryo transfers
D. Accepting childlessness as a lifestyle may also be necessary; support groups (e.g., Resolve) may be helpful.

Nursing Interventions

A. Assist with assessment including a complete history, physical exam, lab work, and tests for both partners.
B. Monitor psychologic reaction to infertility.
C. Support couple through procedures and tests.

D. Identify any existing abnormalities and provide couple with information about their condition(s).

E. Help couple acknowledge and express their feelings both separately and together.

Control of Fertility

Voluntary prevention of conception through various means, some of which employ devices or medications.

Methods of Conception Control

A. Natural methods
   1. Natural family planning
      a. Periodic abstinence from intercourse when ovulating
      b. Uses calculations intended to identify those days of the menstrual cycle when coitus is avoided.
         1) basal body temperature: identification of temperature drop before ovulation, then rise past ovulation; identifies days on which coitus is avoided to avoid conception.
         2) cervical mucus method: identification of changes in cervical mucus; when affected by estrogen and most conducive to penetration by sperm, cervical mucus is clear, stretchy, and slippery; when influenced by progesterone, cervical mucus is thick, cloudy, and sticky and does not allow sperm passage; coitus is avoided during days of estrogen-influenced mucus.
         3) sympto-thermal: combination of basal body temperature and cervical mucus method to increase effectiveness
   2. Coitus interruptus
      a. Withdrawal of the penis from the vagina before ejaculation.
      b. Not very safe; pre-ejaculatory fluids from Cowper's glands may contain live, motile sperm.
      c. Demands precise male control.

B. Chemical barriers
   1. Use of foams, creams, jellies, and vaginal suppositories designed to destroy the sperm or limit their motility
   2. Available without a prescription, widely used, especially in conjunction with the diaphragm and the condom
   3. Need to be placed in the vagina immediately before each act of intercourse; messy
   4. Some people may have allergic reaction to the chemicals

C. Mechanical barriers: diaphragm, condom, cervical cap, contraceptive sponge
   1. Diaphragm: shallow rubber dome fits over cervix, blocking passage of sperm through cervix
      a. Efficiency increased by use of chemical barrier as lubricant

   b. Woman needs to be measured for diaphragm, and refitted after childbirth or weight gain/loss of 10 lb
   c. Device needs to be left in place 6-8 hours after intercourse.
   d. Woman needs to practice insertion and removal, and to be taught how to check for holes in diaphragm, store in cool place.
2. Condom: thin stretchable rubber sheath worn over penis during intercourse
   a. Widely available without prescription
   b. Applied with room at tip to accommodate ejaculate
   c. Applied to erect penis before vaginal penetration
   d. Man is instructed to hold on to rim of condom as he withdraws from female to prevent spilling semen.
3. Cervical cap: cup-shaped device that is placed over cervical os and held in place by suction.
   a. four sizes; client needs to be fitted
   b. women need to practice insertion and removal
   c. spermicidals increase effectiveness
   d. may be left in place for up to 24 hours
4. Contraceptive sponge: small, soft insert, with indentation on one side to fit over cervix; contains spermicide
   a. moistened with water and inserted with indentation snugly against cervix
   b. may be left in place up to 24 hours
   c. no professional fitting required
   d. may also protect against STDs
   e. should not be used by women with history of toxic shock syndrome
   f. problems include cost, difficulty in removal, and irritation
D. Hormone therapy (oral contraceptives, birth control pills)
1. Ingestion of estrogen and progesterone on a specific schedule to prevent the release of FSH and LH, thus preventing ovulation and pregnancy.
2. Causes additional tubal, endometrial, and cervical mucus changes.
3. Available in combined or sequential types.
4. Usually taken beginning on day 5 of the menstrual cycle through day 25, then discontinued.
5. Withdrawal bleeding occurs within 2-3 days.
6. Contraindications
   a. History of hypertension or vascular disorders
   b. Age over 35
   c. Cigarette smoking (heavy)
7. Women using oral contraceptives need to be sure to get sufficient amounts of vitamin B as metabolism of this vitamin is affected.
8. Minor side effects may include
   a. Weight gain
   b. Breast changes

     c. Headaches

     d. Vaginal spotting

  9. Report vision changes/disorders immediately.

E. Intrauterine devices (IUD)
1. Placement of plastic or nonreactive device into uterine cavity
2. Mode of action thought to be the creation of a sterile endometrial inflammation, discourages implantation (nidation).
3. Does not affect ovulation or conception.
4. Device is inserted during or just after menstruation, while cervix is slightly open.
5. May cause cramping or heavy bleeding during menses for several months after insertion.
6. Tail of IUD hangs into vagina through cervix; woman taught to feel for it before intercourse and after each menses.
7. A distinct disadvantage is the increased risk of pelvic infection (PID) with use of IUD.

F. Surgical sterilization
1. Bilateral tubal ligation in the female to prevent the passage of ova.
2. Bilateral vasectomy in the male to prevent the passage of sperm.
3. Both of these operations should be considered permanent.
4. Female will still menstruate but will not conceive.
5. Male will be incapable of fertilizing his partner after all viable sperm ejaculated from vas deferens (6 weeks or 10 ejaculations).
6. There should be no effect on male capacity for erection or penetration.
7. Hysterectomy also causes permanent sterility in the female.

G. Steroid implants: approved in 1990 by FDA; biodegradable rods containing sustained-release, low-dose progesterone. Inhibits LH (luteinizing hormone) release necessary for ovulation. Effective over 5-year time frame. Need minor surgical procedure for insertion and removal. Removal causes total reversibility of effect.

H. Injectable progestin-same action as G; lasts 3 months

Nursing Responsibilities in Control of Fertility

A. Assess previous experience of couple or individual.
B. Obtain health history and perform physical examination.
C. Identify present needs for contraception.
D. Determine motivation regarding contraception.
E. Assist the client/couple in receiving information desired; advise about the various methods available.
F. Ensure that client/couple selects method best suited to their needs.
1. Support choice of client/couple as right for them.
2. Provide time for practice with method chosen, if applicable.
3. Instruct in side effects/potential complications.
G. Encourage expression of feelings about contraception.

Termination of Pregnancy

General Information

A. Deliberate interruption of a pregnancy in a pre-viable time. Legal in all states since Supreme Court ruling of January 1973, as follows
   1. First trimester: determined by pregnant woman and her physician.
   2. Second trimester: determined by pregnant woman and her physician; state can regulate the circumstances to ensure safety.
   3. Third trimester: conditions determined by state law.
B. Indications may be physical or psychologic, socioeconomic or genetic.
C. Techniques vary according to trimester.
   1. First trimester: *vacuum extraction* or *dilatation and curettage (D&C)*
      a. Cervix dilated
      b. Products of conception either aspirated or scraped out
      c. Procedure is short, usually well tolerated by client, and has few complications.
   2. Second trimester
      a. *Saline abortion*
         1) amniotic fluid aspirated from uterus, replaced with same amount 20% saline solution.
         2) contractions begin in 12-24 hours; may be induced by oxytocin (Pitocin)
         3) client is hospitalized; infection or hypernatremia possible complications
      b. *Prostaglandins*
         1) injection of prostaglandin into uterus
         2) contractions initiated in under 1 hour
         3) side effects may include nausea and vomiting
      c. *Hysterotomy*
         1) incision into uterus to remove fetus.
         2) may also be used for sterilization.
         3) client is hospitalized.
         4) care is similar to that for cesarean birth.
   3. Third trimester: same as second trimester, if permitted by state law.

Assessment

A. Vaginal bleeding
B. Vital signs
C. Excessive cramping

Analysis

A. Risk for deficient fluid volume
B. Risk for injury
C. Deficient knowledge

Planning and Implementation

A. Goals
   1. Recovery from procedure will be free from complications.
   2. Client will be supported in her decision.
B. Interventions
   1. Explain procedure to client.
   2. Administer medications as ordered.
   3. Assist with procedure as needed.
   4. Monitor client carefully during procedure.
   5. Monitor client postprocedure.
   6. Administer postprocedure medications as ordered (analgesics, antibiotics, oxytocins, RhoGam if mother Rh negative).
   7. Provide contraceptive information as appropriate.

Evaluation

A. Procedure tolerated without complications; vital signs stable, no hemorrhage, products of conception evacuated, no infection
B. Client supported through procedure; emotionally stable

■ MENSTRUAL DISORDERS

Menstruation is the periodic shedding of the endometrium when there has been no conception. Onset is menarche (age 11-14); cessation is menopause (average age 50).

Assessment

A. Menstrual cycle for symptoms and pattern
B. Client discomfort with cycles
C. Knowledge base about menses

Analysis

A. Deficient knowledge
B. Ineffective health maintenance

Planning and Implementation

A. Goals
   1. Client will receive necessary information.
   2. Client will choose treatment/options best to suited her needs.
B. Interventions
   1. Explain menstrual physiology to client.
   2. Explain options for treatment to client.
   3. Provide time for questions.
   4. Reinforce good menstrual hygiene.
   5. Administer medications if ordered.

NURSING ALERT

B lood loss may be considered significant if the client is changing her pad or tampon every 1–2 hours.

Evaluation

Client demonstrates knowledge of condition and treatment options.

Specific Disorders

Dysmenorrhea

A. Pain associated with menstruation
B. Usually associated with ovulatory cycles; absent when ovulation suppressed
C. Intensified by stress, cultural factors, and presence of an IUD
D. High levels of prostaglandins found in menstrual flow of women with dysmenorrhea
E. Treatment my include rest, application of heat, distraction, exercise, analgesia (especially anti-prostaglandins: NSAIDs)

Amenorrhea

A. Absence of menstruation.
B. Possibly caused by underlying abnormality of endocrine system, rapid weight loss, or strenuous exercise.
C. Treatment is individualized by cause.

Menorrhagia

A. Excessive menstrual flow
B. Possibly caused by endocrine imbalance, uterine tumors, infection
C. Treatment individualized by cause

Metrorrhagia

A. Intercyclic bleeding
B. Frequently the result of a disease process
C. Treatment individualized by cause

Endometriosis

A. Endometrial tissue is found outside the uterus, attached to the ovaries, colon, round ligaments, etc.
B. This tissue reacts to the endocrine stimulation cycle as does the intrauterine endometrium, resulting in inflammation of the extrauterine sites, with pain and fibrosis/scar tissue formation as the eventual result.

C. Actual cause is unknown.

D. May cause dysmenorrhea, dyspareunia, and infertility.

E. Treatment may include the use of oral contraceptives to minimize endometrial buildup or medications to suppress menstruation (Danocrine, Synarel).

F. Pregnancy and lactation may also be recommended as means to suppress menstruation.

G. Surgical intervention (removal of endometrial implants) may be helpful.

H. Hysterectomy and salpingo-oophorectomy are curative.

■ INFECTIOUS DISORDERS

Sexually Transmitted Diseases (STD)

Infections occurring predominantly in the genital area and spread by sexual relations.

Assessment

A. Sexual history/social practices

B. Physical examination for signs and symptoms of specific disorder

Analysis

A. Deficient knowledge

B. Risk for injury

C. Ineffective health maintenance

Planning and Implementation

A. Goals
    1. Disease process will be identified and treated.
    2. Affected others will be identified and treated.
    3. Complications will be prevented.

B. Interventions
    1. Collect specimens for tests.
    2. Implement isolation technique if indicated.
    3. Teach transmission/prevention techniques.
    4. Assist in case finding.
    5. Administer medications as ordered.
    6. Inform client of any necessary lifestyle changes.

Evaluation

A. Client receiving treatment appropriate to specific disorder, understands treatment regimen.

B. Client demonstrates knowledge of disease process and transmission.

C. Affected others have been identified and treated.

Specific Disorders

Herpes

A. Genital herpes is caused by herpes simplex virus type 2 (HSV_2).

B. Causes painful vesicles on genitalia, both external and internal.

C. There is no cure.

D. Treatment is symptomatic.

E. If active infection at the end of pregnancy, cesarean birth may be indicated, since virus may be lethal to neonate who cannot localize infection.

F. Recurrences of the condition may be caused by infection, stress, menses.

G. Acyclovir (Zovirax) reduces severity and duration of exacerbation.

Chlamydia

A. Currently most common STD

B. Symptoms similar to gonorrhea (cervical/vaginal discharge) or may be asymptomatic

C. Can be transmitted to fetus at birth, causes neonatal ophthalmia

D. Treated with erythromycin, prophylactic treatment of neonate's eyes

E. If untreated, can lead to pelvic inflammatory disease (PID)

Gonorrhea

A. Caused by *N. gonorrhoeae*.

B. Symptoms may include heavy, purulent vaginal discharge, but often asymptomatic in female.

C. May be passed to fetus at time of birth, causing ophthalmia neonatorum and sepsis.

D. Treatment is penicillin; allergic clients may be treated with erythromycin or (if not pregnant) the cephalosporins.

E. All sexual contacts must be treated as well, to prevent "ping-pong" recurrence.

Syphilis

A. Caused by *Treponema pallidum* (spirochete)

B. Crosses placenta after 16th week of pregnancy to infect fetus.

C. Initial symptoms are chancre and lymph-adenopathy and may disappear without treatment in 4-6 weeks.

D. Secondary symptoms are rash, malaise, and alopecia; these too may disappear in several weeks without treatment.

E. Tertiary syphilis may recur later in life and affect any organ system, especially cardiovascular and neurologic systems.

F. Diagnosis is made by dark-field exam and serologic tests (VDRL).

G. Treatment is penicillin, or erythromycin if penicillin allergy exists.

Other Genital Infections

Cervical and vaginal infections may be caused by agents other than those associated with STDs. For all female clients with a vaginal infection, nursing actions should include teaching good perineal hygiene.

Trichomonas vaginalis

A. Caused by a protozoan
B. Major symptom is profuse foamy white to greenish discharge that is irritating to genitalia.
C. Treatment is metronidazole (Flagyl) for woman and all sexual partners.
D. Treatment lasts 7 days, during which time a condom should be used for intercourse.
E. Alcohol ingestion with Flagyl causes severe gastrointestinal upset.

Candida albicans

A. Caused by a yeast transmitted from GI tract to vagina.
B. Overgrowth may occur in pregnancy, with diabetes, and with steroid or antibiotic therapy.
C. Vaginal examination reveals thick, white, cheesy patches on vaginal walls.
D. Treatment is topical application of clotrimazole (Gyne-Lotrimin), nystatin (Mycostatin), or gentian violet.
E. **Candida albicans** causes thrush in the newborn by direct contact in the birth canal.

Bacterial Vaginitis

A. Caused by other bacteria invading the vagina
B. Foul or fishy-smelling discharge
C. Treatment is specific to causative agent, and usually includes sexual partners for best results

Female Reproductive System Neoplasia

The nursing diagnoses, general goals and interventions, and evaluation for the client with cancer of the reproductive system are similar to those for any client with a diagnosis of cancer. Only nursing care specific to the disorder will be discussed here.

Fibrocystic Breast Disease

A. Most common benign breast lesion.
B. Cyst(s) may be palpated; surgical biopsy indicated for differential diagnosis.
C. Treatment includes surgical removal of cysts, decreasing or removing caffeine from diet, and medication to suppress menses.

Procedure for Breast Self-Examination (BSE)

A. Age: routine BSE should begin as early in a woman's life as possible. Adolescence is not too early.

B. Timing: regularly, on a monthly basis, 3 to 7 days after the end of the menses, when breasts are least likely to be swollen or tender. After menopause, BSE should be done on one particular day/date every month.

C. Procedure

    1. Inspection: stand before mirror and visually inspect with arms at sides; raised over head; hands on hips with muscles tightened; then leaning forward. Assessment should include size, symmetry, shape, direction, color, skin texture and thickness, nipple size and shape, rashes or discharges. Unusual findings should be reported to health care provider.

    2. Palpation: to examine left breast, woman should be lying down, with left hand behind head and small folded towel or pillow under left shoulder. Using flattened fingertips of right hand and a rotary motion, palpate along lines of concentric circles from outer edges of breast to nipple area, or from outer edge to nipple area following wedge or wheel-spoke lines. Also palpate in the left axillary area where multiple lymph nodes are present, as well as a "tail" of breast tissue. The nipple should be gently squeezed to assess for discharges.

        a. To examine right breast, positions are reversed.

        b. Palpation activities are repeated for each breast with the woman in the sitting position.

        c. Unusual findings are reported to the health care provider.

        d. Breast self-examination (BSE) and mammograms as indicated by age and risk are primary screening tools.

Breast Cancer

A. General information

    1. Most common neoplasm in women

    2. Leading cause of death in women age 40–44

B. Medical management

    1. Usually surgical excision; options are simple lumpectomy, simple mastectomy, modified radical mastectomy, and radical mastectomy.

    2. Adjuvant treatment with chemotherapy, radiation, and hormone therapy.

C. Assessment findings

    1. Palpation of lump (upper outer quadrant most frequent site) usually first symptom

    2. Skin of breast dimpled

    3. Nipple discharge

    4. Asymmetry of breasts

    5. Surgical biopsy provides definitive diagnosis

D. Nursing interventions
   1. Assess breasts for early identification and treatment.
   2. Support client through recommended/chosen treatment.
   3. Prepare client for mastectomy if necessary.

Mastectomy

A. General information
   1. Lumpectomy: removal of lump and surrounding breast tissue; lymph nodes biopsied.
   2. Simple mastectomy: removal of breast only, lymph nodes biopsied.
   3. Radical mastectomy: removal of breast, muscle layer down to chest wall, and axillary lymph nodes.
B. Nursing interventions
   1. Provide routine pre- and post-op care.
   2. Elevate client's arm on operative side on pillows to minimize edema.
   3. Do not use arm on affected side for blood pressure measurements, IVs, or injections.
   4. Turn only to back and unaffected side.
   5. Monitor client for bleeding, check under her.
   6. Begin range-of-motion exercises immediately on unaffected side.
   7. Start with simple movements on affected side: fingers and hands first, then wrist, elbow, and shoulder movements.
   8. Make abduction the last movement.
   9. Coordinate physical therapy if ordered.
   10. Teach client about any necessary life-style changes (special care of arm on affected side, monthly breast self-examination on remaining breast, use of prosthesis).
   11. Encourage/arrange visit from support group member.
C. Medical therapy
   1. Hormonal therapy: tamoxifen, anti-estrogen effect.
   2. Chemotherapy
   3. Radiation
   4. Chemotherapy and radiation used with lumpectomy

Cancer of the Cervix

A. Detected by Pap smear, followed by tissue biopsy.
   1. Class I - normal pap smear
   2. Class II - atypical cells
   3. Class III - moderate dysplasia
   4. Class IV - severe dysplasia, cancer-in-situ
   5. Class V - Squamous cell carcinoma, invasive Ca
B. Preinvasive conditions may be treated by cryosurgery, laser surgery, cervical conization, or hysterectomy.

NURSING ALERT

If a myectomy has been preformed, pregnancy is still possible.

C. Invasive conditions are treated by radium therapy and radical hysterectomy.

Cancer of the Uterus

A. May affect endometrium or fundus/corpus risk increased by unopposed estrogen.
B. Cardinal symptom: abnormal uterine bleeding, either pre- or postmenopause
C. Diagnosis: by endometrial biopsy or fractional curettage; cells washed from uterus under pressure may also be used for diagnosis
D. Usual intervention: total hysterectomy and bilateral salpingo-oophorectomy
E. Radium therapy and chemotherapy may also be used.

Cancer of the Ovary

A. Etiology unknown.
B. Few early symptoms; palpation of ovarian mass is usual first finding.
C. Treatment of choice is surgical removal with total hysterectomy and bilateral salpingo-oophorectomy.
D. Chemotherapy may be used as adjuvant therapy.

Cancer of the Vulva

A. Begins as small, pruritic lesions
B. Diagnosed by biopsy
C. Treatment is either local excision or radical vulvectomy (removal of entire vulva plus superficial and femoral nodes).

Hysterectomy

A. General information
   1. Total hysterectomy: removal of uterine body and cervix only
   2. Subtotal hysterectomy: removal of uterine body leaving cervix in place (seldom performed)
   3. Total abdominal hysterectomy with bilateral salpingo-oophorectomy (TAH-BSO): removal of uterine body, cervix, both ovaries, and both fallopian tubes

CLIENT TEACHING CHECKLIST

Instruct the client regarding:

- The type of surgery and follow-up care
- The need for hormone replacement , if indicated
- Eating a well-balanced diet
- Avoiding heavy lifting for 6 weeks
- Avoiding aerobic activity
- Avoiding vaginal and rectal intrusions
- Reporting any fresh bleeding

4. Radical hysterectomy: removal of uterine body, cervix, connective tissue, part of vagina, and pelvic lymph nodes

B. Nursing interventions
   1. Institute routine pre- and post-op care.
   2. Assess for hemorrhage, infection, or other postsurgical complications (e.g., paralytic ileus, thrombophlebitis, pneumonia).
   3. Support woman and family through procedure, encourage expression of feelings and reactions to procedure.
   4. Explain implications of hysterectomy.
      a. No further menses.
      b. If ovaries also removed, will have menopause and may need estrogen replacement therapy.
   5. Allow woman (and partner) to verbalize concerns about sexuality postsurgery.
   6. Provide discharge teaching.

Menopause

The time in a woman's life when menstruation ceases. Fertility usually ceases, and symptoms associated with changing hormone levels may occur. Reactions to menopause may be influenced by culture, age at menopause, reproductive and menstrual history, and complications.

Assessment Findings

A. Symptoms related to hormone changes
   1. Vasomotor instability (hot flashes and night sweats)
   2. Emotional disturbances (mood swings, irritability, depression), fatigue, and headache

B. Physical changes include
   1. Atrophy of genitalia

NURSING ALERT

A positive indicator of the onset of menopause is an FSH level higher than 40 mIU/ml and a low serum estradiol level.

2. Dyspareunia
3. Urinary changes (frequency/stress incontinence)
4. Constipation
5. Possibly uterine prolapse

Interventions

A. Estrogen replacement therapy (ERT)
   1. Used to control symptoms, especially vasomotor instability and vaginal atrophy, and to prevent osteoporosis
   2. Women with family histories of breast or uterine cancer, hypertension, thrombophlebitis, or cardiac dysfunction are not good candidates for ERT.
   3. Women may need information about contraception, as ovulation and ability to conceive may continue for up to 12 months after menses cease.
   4. Sold under many pharmaceutical trade names; may be taken orally, or applied transdermally (patch).
   5. Women who still have a uterus must take progesterone to decrease risk of endometrial cancer. New studies have shown long-term use carries serious risk.
B. Alternatives to ERT include
   1. Vitamin E: from dietary sources and supplements
   2. Herbs: varied relief with combinations of roots and herbs, such as licorice and dandelion
   3. Other medications: Bellergal (phenobarbital, ergotamine tartrate, and belladonna)
   4. Kegel exercises for genital atrophy: alternating constriction and relaxation of pubococcygeal muscles (muscles controlling the flow of urine) done at least three times/day
   5. Vaginal lubricants for genital atrophy: water-soluble lubricants can diminish dyspareunia
   6. Maintenance of good hydration: at least 8 glasses of water/day
   7. Good perineal hygiene

Complications of Menopause

Osteoporosis

A. Increased porosity of the bone, with increased incidence of spontaneous fractures.

B. Other symptoms in the postmenopausal woman include loss of height, back pain, and dowager's hump.

C. Diagnosis by X-ray is not possible until more than 50% of bone mass has already been lost.

D. Decreased bone porosity is inextricably linked with lowered levels of estrogen in the postmenopausal woman. Estrogen plays a part in the absorption of calcium and the stimulation of osteoclasts (new-bone-forming cells).

E. Treatment includes
1. ERT unless contraindicated
2. Supplemental calcium to slow the osteoporotic process (1 g taken daily at HS)
3. Increased fluid intake (2–3 liters/day will help avoid formation of calculi)
4. High-calcium/high-phosphorus diet with avoidance of excess protein
5. Some exercise on a regular basis

F. Prevention includes
1. Not smoking
2. Regular weight-bearing exercise
3. Good nutrition, including sources of calcium and vitamin D
4. Minimal use or exclusion of alcohol
5. Regular physical examination

Cystocele/Rectocele

A. Herniations of the anterior and posterior (respectively) walls of the vagina.

B. Usually the sequelae of childbirth injuries.

C. Herniation allows the bulging of the bladder and the rectum into the vagina.

D. Treatment is surgical repair of these conditions: anterior and posterior *colporrhaphy*.

Prolapse of the Uterus

A. Usually the result of childbirth injuries or relaxation of the cardinal ligaments.

B. Allows the uterus to sag backward and downward into the vagina, or outside the body completely.

C. Vaginal hysterectomy is the preferred surgical intervention.

D. If condition does not warrant surgery, the insertion of a *pessary* (supportive device) will help to support and stabilize the uterus.

REVIEW QUESTIONS

1. In collecting data for a health history of an infertility client, which of the following findings is most important?

   1. She is 5 ft 8 in tall and weighs 105 lb.
   2. She has never used any form of contraception.
   3. She has been married for 3 years.
   4. She has no brothers or sisters.

2. The teaching plan for a woman who has just been fitted with her first diaphragm must include

   1. specific amount of spermicide to be used with diaphragm.
   2. insertion at least 8 hours before intercourse.
   3. specific cleaning techniques.
   4. storage in the refrigerator.

3. A 64-year-old postmenopausal woman takes calcium supplements on a daily basis. She can reduce the danger of renal calculi by the simple action of

   1. chewing her calcium tablets rather than swallowing them whole.
   2. swallowing her calcium tablets with cranberry juice.
   3. eliminating other sources of calcium from her diet.
   4. drinking 2–3 quarts of water daily.

4. A 57-year-old woman is having a routine physical exam. Which of the following assessments would yield critical information as to her postmenopausal status?

   1. Asking about weight loss of more than 5 lb in the last year.
   2. Asking about her nightly sleep patterns.
   3. Asking about her cultural background.
   4. Asking about her last pregnancy.

5. A 46-year-old woman is admitted to the hospital for a panhysterectomy. Which nursing strategy should be included in the nursing care plan to meet her body-image perception changes?

   1. Allowing her time to work out her feelings on her own.
   2. Discouraging fears about weight gain.
   3. Helping her verbalize her concerns about her femininity.
   4. Insisting that she look at the scar.

6. Following a panhysterectomy, the woman is placed on estrogen replacement therapy. The primary purpose of estrogen replacement therapy following surgical menopause is to prevent
   1. arthritis.
   2. pregnancy.
   3. breast cancer.
   4. vasomotor instability.

7. A 39-year-old woman has advanced cancer of the breast. She is admitted to the medical unit for nutritional evaluation. She weighs 101 lb and is 5 ft 8 in tall. She is started on leucovorin (Wellcovorin). Assessment of her nutritional health would include all the following except
   1. a diet history.
   2. anthropometric measurements.
   3. food preferences.
   4. serum protein studies.

8. The nurse's primary role relating to sexually transmitted disease is
   1. case reporting.
   2. sexual counseling.
   3. diagnosis and treatment.
   4. recognizing symptoms and teaching clients.

9. A 17-year-old comes to the local health clinic because her boyfriend was recently diagnosed as having gonorrhea. She asks the nurse what would have happened to her if she had gone without treatment. The nurse explains that the possible consequences of lack of treatment could result in
   1. disseminated systemic infections.
   2. minor problems such as skin rashes.
   3. the need for delivery by cesarean section.
   4. sterility, birth defects, and miscarriage.

10. Several adolescent girls are discussing sexual activity with the nurse at the STD clinic. Which comment indicates to the nurse that the client has not understood the teaching regarding safe sexual practices?
    1. "We use KY jelly on condoms."
    2. "I douche after intercourse."
    3. "I shower with my boyfriend."
    4. "We use condoms and birth control pills."

11. When discussing safe sex, which information about the use of condoms would be most helpful?

    1. Lambskin condoms do not interfere with sensation.
    2. Latex condoms help prevent the transmission of germs.
    3. Condoms are often inconvenient and unnecessary.
    4. Condoms prevent STDs but they are a poor choice for birth control.

12. A couple have come to your clinic because they have not been able to achieve a pregnancy after trying for 2 years without using any form of birth control. Which of the following tests could determine that the woman is ovulating regularly?

    1. Hysterosalpingogram.
    2. Serial basal body temperature graph.
    3. Postcoital test.
    4. Semen analysis.

13. A woman is preparing to take Clomid to induce ovulation so she can have an in vitro fertilization. She asks if she should expect any side effects from the drug. Your *best* answer should include which of the following?

    1. Weight gain with increased appetite and constipation.
    2. Tingling of the hands and feet.
    3. Alopecia (hair loss).
    4. Stuffy nose and cold-like symptoms.

14. A couple have been using a diaphragm for contraception. Which of the following statements indicates they are using it correctly?

    1. "We use K-Y jelly around the rim to help with insertion."
    2. "I wash the diaphragm each time and hold it up to the light to look for any holes."
    3. "I take the diaphragm out about 1 hour after intercourse because it feels funny."
    4. "I douche right away after intercourse."

15. A 25-year-old wishes to take oral contraceptives. When taking her history, which of the following questions would determine if she is an appropriate candidate for this form of birth control?

    1. "Do you currently smoke cigarettes and, if so, how many?"
    2. "Have you had any recent weight gain or loss?"
    3. "Do you douche regularly after intercourse?"
    4. "Is there any family history of kidney or gallbladder disease?"

16. A woman who is 18 weeks pregnant is scheduled for a saline injection to terminate her pregnancy. She asks the nurse what she should expect. Your *best* answer is,

   1. "Contractions will begin immediately after the instillation of saline and will be mild."

   2. "An amniocentesis will be performed with amniotic fluid removal and saline replacement."

   3. "A tube will be inserted through the cervix and warm saline will be administered by continuous drip."

   4. "The baby will be born alive but will die a short time later."

17. A woman comes to the office complaining of the following symptoms: fatigue, weight gain, pelvic pain related to menstruation, heartburn, and constipation. Which of the above symptoms might indicate a diagnosis of endometriosis?

   1. Weight gain and fatigue.

   2. Heartburn.

   3. Constipation.

   4. Pelvic pain related to menstruation.

18. A woman has been diagnosed with *Candida albicans*. Which of the following types of vaginal discharge would you expect to find?

   1. Thin, greenish yellow with a foul odor.

   2. Either a yellowish discharge or none at all.

   3. Thick and white, like cottage cheese.

   4. Thin, grayish white with a fishy odor.

19. A woman has just been diagnosed with genital herpes for the first time. You can expect which of the following treatments to be part of her plan of care?

   1. Vaginal soaks with saline to keep the area moist.

   2. Acyclovir 200 mg 5 times daily for 7-10 days.

   3. Ceftriaxone 125 mg IM times 1 dose.

   4. Topical application of podophyllin to the lesions.

20. A woman is 10 weeks pregnant and tested positive for syphilis but has no symptoms. She asks you why she needs to be treated since she feels fine? Your *best* response to her would include which of the following?

   1. "Syphilis can be transmitted to the baby and may cause it to die before birth if you are not treated."

   2. "If you do not receive treatment before the baby is born, your baby could become blind."

3. "If syphilis is untreated, the baby may be mentally retarded at birth."

4. "Syphilis may cause your baby to have a heart problem when it is born."

21. A woman has been diagnosed with fibrocystic breast disease. Which of the following should be included in the teaching plan for her?

   1. Limiting breast self-examinations to every 3 months because it may be painful.

   2. Wearing a bra as little as possible because pressure on the breast may be painful.

   3. Limiting caffeine and salt intake.

   4. Using heat to the tender areas of the breast.

22. The local YWCA is having a series of seminars on health-related topics. You are invited to discuss breast self-examination (BSE) with the group. Which of the following would be appropriate to teach regarding when BSE should be performed by women of reproductive age?

   1. At the end of each menstrual cycle.

   2. At the beginning of each menstrual cycle.

   3. About 7–10 days after the beginning of each menstrual cycle.

   4. About 7–10 days before the end of the menstrual cycle.

23. You have been discussing breast self-examination (BSE) with a woman. Which of the following statements would *best* indicate she is doing BSE correctly?

   1. "I begin to examine my breasts by placing the palm of my right hand on the nipple of the left breast."

   2. "I don't like to press very hard because my breasts are very tender."

   3. "I use the tips of the middle three fingers of each hand to feel each breast."

   4. "I feel for lumps in my breasts standing in front of a mirror."

24. A 32-year-old had a simple mastectomy this morning. Which of the following should be included in your plan for her care?

   1. Complete bed rest for the first 24 hours.

   2. NPO with IV fluids for the first 48 hours.

   3. Positioning on the operative side for the first 24 hours.

   4. Keep patient-controlled anesthesia (PCA) controller within easy reach for the first 48 hours.

25. The nurse is teaching a woman who had a simple mastectomy. Which of the following would be appropriate to tell her?

1. She should wait to be fitted for a permanent prosthesis until the wound is completely healed.

2. Since she had a simple mastectomy, she will probably not feel the need to attend Reach for Recovery meetings.

3. She will have very little pain and the incision will heal very quickly.

4. She should refrain from seeking male companionship since she will be seen as less than a woman.

26. A group of women have gathered at the local library for a series of seminars about women's health issues. In discussing cancer of the cervix, which of the following would be accurate?

   1. This cancer is very rapid growing, so early detection is difficult to achieve.

   2. A cervical biopsy is the screening test of choice for early detection of cervical cancer.

   3. All women have an equal chance to develop cervical cancer because there are no high risk factors.

   4. An annual Pap smear may detect cervical dysplasia, a frequent precursor of cervical cancer.

27. The nurse is talking to a woman who has been diagnosed with cancer of the ovary. She asks you what she could have done so that the cancer would have been found earlier. The best response should include which of the following?

   1. She should have had more frequent, twice a year, Pap smears.

   2. A yearly complete blood count (CBC) could have provided valuable clues to detect ovarian cancer.

   3. Detection of ovarian cancer is easier if a yearly proctoscopy is done.

   4. There is little more she could have done for earlier detection.

28. The nurse is caring for a woman who has had a vaginal hysterectomy and an indwelling Foley catheter. After removal of the catheter, she is unable to void and has little sensation of bladder fullness. She is also constipated and is experiencing some perineal pain. The *most* appropriate nursing diagnosis is altered urinary elimination related to

   1. infection as evidenced by inability to void with frequency and urgency.

   2. retention as evidenced by inability to void and urinary distention.

   3. gastrointestinal functioning as evidenced by inability to void and constipation.

   4. dysuria as evidenced by inability to void and loss of bladder sensation.

29. A 42-year-old had a simple vaginal hysterectomy without oophorectomy due to uterine fibroids. You have completed your discharge teaching and

she is preparing to go home. Which of the following statements indicates she understands the physical changes she will experience?

1. "I hope my husband will still love me since we can't have sexual intercourse anymore."

2. "I was hoping to stop having periods, but I guess that will need to wait a few more years."

3. "It will be so nice to not need to use birth control any more."

4. "I just don't think I will ever feel feminine again since I can no longer experience orgasm."

30. The nurse has been discussing menopause with a 50-year-old woman who is experiencing some bodily changes indicative of the perimenopausal period. Which of the following statements indicates the client understands what is happening to her body?

1. "Even though I am only having periods every few months, I should continue to use birth control until at least 6 months after my periods have stopped."

2. "I am very upset to think that I will continue to have these hot flashes for the rest of my life."

3. "Now that I am an old woman, I guess I'll be sick most of the time, so I should plan to move to a retirement home."

4. "I may continue to bleed on and off throughout the next 25 years."

31. A 55-year-old woman who has ceased having menses has a family history of osteoporosis and increasing cholesterol levels over the past several years. Hormone replacement therapy (HRT) has been prescribed with estrogen and progesterone. She asks you why she should take the pills since she feels quite well. The nurse's answer would be

1. HRT is thought to help protect women from heart disease and osteoporosis.

2. HRT will help to reestablish the menstrual cycle, thus providing natural protection against heart disease and osteoporosis.

3. even though she feels well now, she will soon begin having major health problems and HRT will protect her against those problems.

4. she will be protected from breast cancer by HRT.

ANSWERS AND RATIONALES

1. 1. Because of the complex interaction between the hypothalamus, the ovary, and the amount of body fat, women who are underweight or who engage in strenuous physical activity over prolonged periods of time may experience changes in their menstrual cycle and their fertility.

2. 3. The client must be instructed to clean the diaphragm with mild, plain soap, and warm water; dust it lightly with cornstarch; and store it in a cool, dry place. She should also be instructed to check it regularly for perforations or defects.

3. 4. The ingestion of sufficient amounts of water by a woman taking calcium supplements is important to prevent renal calculi.

4. 2. Postmenopausal women who are experiencing vasomotor instability may have night sweats and interrupted sleep.

5. 3. Loss of the organs of reproduction are often equated with a loss of femininity. The client should be encouraged to explore her feelings and to adapt to body changes.

6. 4. Low-dose estrogen therapy is used to relieve the vasomotor symptoms of menopausal women.

7. 3. Food preferences are considered when planning a program to meet the client's nutritional requirement after the nutritional assessment has been completed.

8. 4. Early recognition of sexually transmitted diseases (STDs) reduces the risk of serious sequelae. The primary role of the nurse is to recognize symptoms of STDs in order to teach clients how to comply with treatment and how to prevent reinfection.

9. 4. Lack of treatment or inadequate treatment of gonorrhea can result in serious sequelae such as sterility, birth defects, and miscarriage. These are the most common complications and the ones most important to discuss.

10. 2. Douching does not protect against infection and damages the natural protective barriers.

11. 2. Condoms can prevent the transmission of many STDs. This information is very important to give.

12. 2. Serial basal body temperature graphs are a baseline for determining when ovulation has taken place during a menstrual cycle. If ovulation has occurred, the temperature will be higher the second half of the cycle and lower the first half.

13. 1. Weight gain associated with increased appetite and constipation are fairly common side effects of Clomid.

14. 2. The diaphragm should be washed and dried and inspected for holes before being put away.

15. 1. Cigarette smoking significantly increases a woman's risk for circulatory complications and may contraindicate oral contraceptive use.

16. 2. The procedure begins with an amniocentesis where amniotic fluid is withdrawn and replaced with saline solution.

17. 4. Pelvic pain related to menstruation is the most common symptom of endometriosis. The pain usually ends following cessation of menses.

18. 3. Thick, white cottage cheese-like discharge is consistent with *Candida albicans.*

19. 2. This is the correct drug and dosage for an initial infection of genital herpes.

20. 1. Syphilis is associated with stillbirth, premature birth, and neonatal death.

21. 3. Most women benefit from caffeine and salt restriction because this reduces fluid retention and increases comfort.

22. 3. The breasts are softer, less tender, and swelling is reduced about a week after the beginning of the menstrual cycle.

23. 3. The ends of the three middle fingers are the most sensitive and should be used for BSE.

24. 4. Adequate pain relief is important and the use of PCA allows the client to control her own pain relief.

25. 1. The incisional site may change with time and healing, so a permanent prosthesis should be purchased only after complete healing has occurred.

26. 4. Cervical dysplasia is frequently a forerunner of cervical cancer and is readily detected by Pap smear; thus follow-up Pap smears allow for early detection and treatment of cervical cancer.

27. 4. Detection of ovarian cancer is very difficult because it gives only vague, subtle symptoms and there are no diagnostic screening tests.

28. 2. Retention of urine is common following vaginal hysterectomy due to stretching of musculature and proximity of the surgery to the bladder and its enervation.

29. 3. After the loss of the uterus, pregnancy is unachievable and birth control is not needed even if the ovaries remain.

30. 1. Even though ovulation is erratic and many periods are anovulatory, birth control should be continued for at least 6 months after the last menses.

31. 1. HRT appears to help protect many women from heart disease and osteoporosis if used with exercise and calcium supplements.

Appendices Table of Contents

Appendix A: Screening Tests in Pregnancy

TEST	RESULTS
Complete Blood Count	
RBC	3.75 million/mm^3 due to hemodilution.
WBC	Rises to 18,000/mm^3 by late pregnancy. Mostly an increase in neutrophils.
Hemoglobin (Hgb)	May decrease to 11.5g/dL later in pregnancy due to hemodilution. Repeat at 28 and 36 weeks.
Hematocrit (Hct)	33% lowest acceptable, due to hemodilution.
Blood Type	A, B, AB, or O
Rh factor	Positive or negative. If negative, do indirect Coomb's test. Check father's Rh.
Coomb's Test	Should remain negative. Retest Rh negative woman at 28 weeks.
Rubella Titer (HAI)	>1:10 indicates immunity, <1:10, immunize after birth of infant.

Continued

176

TEST	RESULTS
Blood Glucose	Should be 60–110 mg/dL. Retest at 24 and 32 weeks.
VDRL or RPR (Syphilis)	Should be negative.

Cervical/Vaginal Culture
  Gonorrhea
  Chlamydia
  Group B
    Streptococcus
	Should be negative.

Hepatitis B Surface Antigen (HB_sAg)	Positive indicates either active hepatitis or carrier state.
Antibody Titer HB_sAg	Positive indicates immunity to hepatitis.
HIV (many states mandate that it be offered)	Should be negative.
Tuberculosis skin tests: Mantoux or Tine	Should be negative. If positive, do chest X-ray.
Urinalysis Color, specific gravity, pH, ketones, albumin, glucose	Same as nonpregnant. Repeat at 28 weeks. Trace of glycosuria may occur in pregnancy.
Alpha-fetoprotein (AFP)	Check with laboratory for normal range for each week of gestation. If elevated, may have neural tube defects. If decreased, may have Down syndrome.

Appendix B: Stages of Fetal Development

STAGE	FETAL DEVELOPMENT
Embryonic or Germinal Stage	
Weeks 1 and 2	Rapid cell division and differentiation. Germinal layers form.
Embryonic Stage	
Week 3*	Primitive nervous system, eyes, ears, and RBCs present. Heart begins to beat on day 21.
Week 4* Wt 0.4 g L 4-6 mm (crown-rump, C-R)	Half the size of a pea. Brain differentiates. Gl tract begins to form. Limb buds appear.

4 weeks

178

STAGE	FETAL DEVELOPMENT
Week 5* L 6-8 mm (C-R)	Cranial nerves present. Muscles innervated.
Week 6* L 10-14 mm (C-R)	Fetal circulation established. Liver produces RBCs. Central autonomic nervous system forms. Primitive kidneys form. Lung buds present. Cartilage forms. Primitive skeleton forms. Muscles differentiate.
Week 7* L 22-28 mm (C-R)	Eyelids form. Palate and tongue form. Stomach formed. Diaphragm formed. Arms and legs move.
Week 8* Wt 2 g L 3 cm (1.2 in) (C-R)	Resembles human being. Eyes moved to face front. Heart development complete. Hands and feet well formed. Bone cells begin replacing cartilage. All body organs have begun forming.
Fetal Stage Week 9	Finger and toenails form. Eyelids fuse shut.
Week 10 Wt 14 g (1/2 oz) L 5-6 cm (2 in) Crown-heel (C-H)	Head growth slows. Islets of Langerhans differentiated. Bone marrow forms, RBCs produced. Bladder sac forms. Kidneys make urine.

8 weeks

Continued

	Week 11	Tooth buds appear. Liver secretes bile. Urinary system functions. Insulin forms in pancreas.
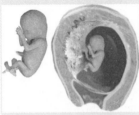 12 weeks	Week 12 Wt 45 g (1.5 oz) L 9 cm (3.5 in) (C–R) 11.5 cm (4.5 in) (C–H)	Lungs take shape. Palate fuses. Heart beat heard with Doppler ultrasound. Ossification established. Swallowing reflex present. External genitalia. Male or female distinguished.
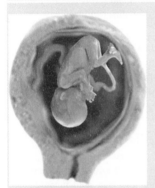 16 weeks	**Second Trimester** Week 16 Wt 200 g (7 oz) L 13.5 cm (5.5 in) (C–R) 15 cm (6 in) (C–H)	Meconium forms in bowels. Scalp hair appears. Frequent fetal movement. Skin thin. Sensitive to light. 200 mL amniotic fluid. (Amniocentesis possible.)
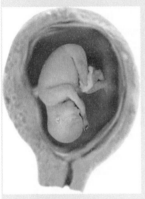 20 weeks	Week 20 Wt 435 g (15 oz) L 19 cm (7.5 in) (C–R) 25 cm (10 in) (C–H)	Myelination of spinal cord begins. Peristalsis begins. Lanugo covers body. Vernix caseosa covers body. Brown fat deposits begun. Sucks and swallows amniotic fluid. Hearbeat heard with fetoscope. Hands can grasp. Regular schedule of sucking, kicking, and sleeping.

	STAGE	FETAL DEVELOPMENT
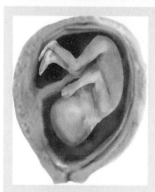 24 weeks	Week 24 Wt 780 g (1 lb, 12 oz) L 23 cm (9 in) (C-R) 28 cm (11 in) (C-H)	Alveoli present in lungs, begin producing surfactant. Eyes completely formed. Eyelashes and eyebrows appear. Many reflexes appear. Chance of survival if born now.
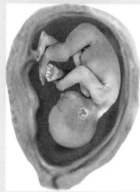 28 weeks	**Third Trimester** Week 28 Wt 1200 g (2 lb, 10 oz) L 28 cm (11 in) (C-R) 35 cm (14 in) (C-H) Eyelids open and close.	Subcutaneous fat deposits begun. Lanugo begins to disappear. Nails appear. Testes begin to descend.
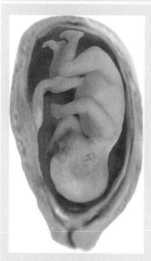 32 weeks	Week 32 Wt 2,000 g (4 lb, 6.5 oz) L 31 cm (12 in) (C-R) 41 cm (16 in) (C-H)	More reflexes present. CNS directs rhythmic breathing movements. CNS partially controls body temperature. Begins storing iron, calcium, phosphorus. Ratio of the lung surfactants lecithin and sphingomyelin (L/S) is 1.2:2.

Continued

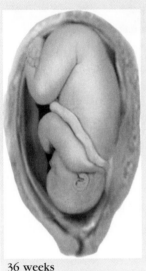

36 weeks

Week 36	A few creases on soles of feet.
Wt 2,500–2.750 g (5 lb, 8 oz)	Skin less wrinkled. Fingernails reach fingertips.
L 35 cm (14 in) (C-R) 48 cm (19 in) (C-H)	Sleep-wake cycle fairly definite. Transfer of maternal antibodies.

| Week 38 | L/S ratio 2:1 |

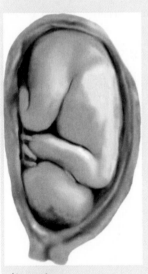

40 weeks

Week 40	Lanugo only on shoulders and upper back.
Wt 3,000–3,600 g (6 lb, 10 oz-7 lb, 15 oz)	Creases cover soles. Vernix mainly in folds of skin.
L 50 cm (20 in) (C-H)	Ear cartilage firm. Less active, limited space. Ready to be born.

*Vulnerable to teratogenic effects.

Appendix C: Specific Educational Content For Each Trimester

■ FIRST TRIMESTER

Knowledge of the Pregnancy

- Anatomy and physiology of pregnancy
- Physical and emotional changes related to pregnancy
- Fetal development
- Importance of prenatal care
- Diagnostic tests, such as chorionic villus sampling, amniocentesis, and ultrasonography
- Warning signs of complications
- Dangers of substance abuse and exposure to toxins and teratogenic hazards

Management of Pregnancy

- Morning sickness
- Sleep disturbances
- Libido changes
- Urinary frequency
- Fatigue
- Emotional lability

Relaxation Techniques

- Awareness of the stress response: breathing patterns, muscle tension, and other physical symptoms of stress in contrast with relaxation
- Awareness of stimuli for tension and relaxation
- Introduction to relaxation techniques
- Slow-paced breathing
- Body awareness

Exercise and Nutrition
- Nutritional needs
- Vitamin supplements
- Exercise
- Body mechanics
- Stretching
- Kegel exercises
- Pelvic tilt exercises
- Toning and aerobic exercises

Family Adaptation
- Choices of provider and birth setting
- Response to emotional and physical changes of pregnancy
- Sexuality
- Infant feeding method
- Exploring maternal and paternal roles
- Communication skills to discuss adaptive changes in the family
- Introduction of discussion of financial and spatial family adaptation to the expanding family

■ SECOND TRIMESTER

Builds on previous teaching or incorporates previous trimester teaching if necessary

Knowledge of Pregnancy
- Physiologic changes of pregnancy
- Fetal development and characteristics
- Fetal movement
- Review of warning signs and complications

Management of Pregnancy
- Management of heartburn, back pain, and discomforts
- Changes in body and body image
- Comfort and hygiene measures

Relaxation Techniques
- Explore and identify techniques, such as imagery, massage, music, touch, visualization, and so on
- Work together as a couple (client and support person) to elicit relaxation to stimuli
- Practice slow-paced breathing, modified-paced breathing, and patterned-paced breathing

Exercise and Nutrition

- Continue good nutrition and monitor weight gain
- Increase repetitions of exercise
- Modify activity related to physical changes

Family Adaptation

- Identity of the fetus as a separate individual and building maternal-fetal attachment
- Financial considerations; may include a discussion of working or career in relation to the pregnancy
- Paternal concerns: role in labor, role as father, financial concerns, and provision of safety for the mother and fetus
- Sibling preparation
- Preparation of the home for the infant
- Discussion of feeding choices for the infant
- Selection of a pediatric provider

■ THIRD TRIMESTER

Often the time for formal classes and need to include all of the above if not already covered

Knowledge of Pregnancy

- Anatomy and physiology of late pregnancy
- Mechanisms and signs of labor
- Additional testing or medical information related to specific conditions
- Medications and anesthesia
- Policies and practices of the facility chosen for delivery
- Postdelivery physical and emotional changes
- Signs and symptoms of labor
- Warning signs of complications
- Progress of labor

Management of Pregnancy

- Preparation for labor
- Comfort measures
- Sleep patterns

Relaxation Techniques

- Practice relaxation techniques
- Practice all methods of breathing for labor
- Practice additional relaxation techniques

Exercise and Nutrition
- Continue good eating patterns
- Monitor appropriate weight gain
- Watch body mechanics, safety, and comfort
- Prepare for delivery: tailor sitting, pelvic tilt, and Kegel exercises
- Perform walking and other conditioning exercises
- Introduce postpartum exercise

Family Adaptation
- Rehearse preparation for delivery and role of support person
- Evaluate family and extended family's preparation for birth
- Discuss normal appearance, care, and feeding of the infant
- Discuss breast-feeding techniques and preparation
- Discuss parental roles
- Discuss sexual adjustment

Appendix D: Common Nursing Diagnoses, Causes, and Outcomes

NURSING DIAGNOSIS	CAUSE	EXPECTED OUTCOMES
Risk for (or present) infection	Unsafe sexual practices, preexisting sexually transmitted disease, lack of immunity to childhood diseases that place the fetus at risk, environmental hazards such as parasites	Fetus is protected from infection by immunization maternal antibiotic treatment, maternal safer see practices and lifestyle precautions, and safe for handling and preparation.
Risk for injury (fetal)	Industrial waste, employment conditions that expose pregnant woman to dangerous chemicals or activities	Fetus is protected from injury by removing hazard from environment, protecting pregnant woman from exposure, and modifying of employment or household conditions.
Ineffective tissue perfusion (placental)	Cigarette smoking, cocaine use, stress	Placental perfusion is adequate, as demonstrated appropriate fetal growth and reassuring fetal assessments.
Impaired gas exchange	Cigarette smoking, carbon monoxide exposure,	Fetus demonstrates adequate oxygenation by reactive

Continued

187

(placental-fetal)	maternal anoxia from seizures	nonstress tests and other assessment
		Risk is reduced by reduction in maternal cigarette smoking and maintenance of therapeutic level of anticonvulsants.Common Nursing Diagnoses, Causes, and Outcomes
Delayed growth and development (fetal)	Inadequate nutrition or malformations from chemical or drug exposure	Alterations are diagnosed promptly. Chemical exposures are minimized or eliminated.
		Pregnant woman and family are informed of risks and supported in decision-making.
		Pregnant woman and family have adequate supp and preparation for birth of an infant with possible altered development.
Imbalanced nutrition, less than body requirements	Substance abuse and consequent anorexia, cognitive alterations, lifestyle disruption	Pregnant woman who abuses substances demonstrates adequate weight gain and fetal growth.
		Adequate support and teaching are provided to re substance abuse and promote healthful lifestyle
Fatigue	Strenuous employment demands	Pregnant woman demonstrates moderation in physical activity and adequate rest periods.
Ineffective role performance	Role burdens (work and home), changing roles	Employment conditions and role expectations are modified to promote prenatal health.

NURSING DIAGNOSIS	CAUSE	EXPECTED OUTCOMES
Fear	Possible birth of damaged infant from exposure to a hazardous substance or infection	Pregnant woman and family report reduction in fear, and demonstrate knowledge of likelihood of fetal harm and measures to minimize fetal damage.
Deficient knowledge	Lack of information about pregnancy, hazards, risk reduction strategies	Pregnant woman and family can state potential risks of their environmental conditions for fetal health, and describe and demonstrate risk reduction strategies.
Ineffective individual and family coping	Substance abuse	Pregnant woman and family demonstrate improved safety in behavior and home management and increased motivation toward healthful behaviors.

Appendix E: NANDA Nursing Diagnoses 2005–2006

Activity Intolerance

Risk for Activity Intolerance

Impaired Adjustment

Ineffective Airway Clearance

Latex Allergy Response

Risk for Latex Allergy Response

Anxiety

Death Anxiety

Risk for Aspiration

Risk for Impaired Parent/Infant/Child Attachment

Autonomic Dysreflexia

Risk for Autonomic Dysreflexia

Disturbed Body Image

Risk for Imbalanced Body Temperature

Bowel Incontinence

Effective Breastfeeding

Ineffective Breastfeeding

Interrupted Breastfeeding

Ineffective Breathing Pattern

Decreased Cardiac Output

Caregiver Role Strain

Risk for Caregiver Role Strain

Impaired Verbal Communication

Readiness for Enhanced Communication

Decisional Conflict (Specify)

Parental Role Conflict

Acute Confusion

Chronic Confusion

Constipation

Perceived Constipation

Risk for Constipation

Defensive Coping

Ineffective Coping

Readiness for Enhanced Coping

Ineffective Community Coping

Readiness for Enhanced Community Coping

Compromised Family Coping

Disabled Family Coping

Readiness for Enhanced Family Coping

Risk for Sudden Infant Death Syndrome

Ineffective Denial

Impaired Dentition

Risk for Delayed Development

190

Diarrhea

Risk for Disuse Syndrome

Deficient Diversional Activity

Energy Field Disturbance

Impaired Environmental Interpretation Syndrome

Adult Failure to Thrive

Risk for Falls

Dysfunctional Family Processes: Alcoholism

Interrupted Family Processes

Readiness for Enhanced Family Processes

Fatigue

Fear

Readiness for Enhanced Fluid Balance

Deficient Fluid Volume

Excess Fluid Volume

Risk for Deficient Fluid Volume

Risk for Imbalanced Fluid Volume

Impaired Gas Exchange

Anticipatory Grieving

Dysfunctional Grieving

Risk for Dysfunctional Grieving

Delayed Growth and Development

Risk for Disproportionate Growth

Ineffective Health Maintenance

Health-Seeking Behaviors (Specify)

Impaired Home Maintenance

Hopelessness

Hyperthermia

Hypothermia

Disturbed Personal Identity

Functional Urinary Incontinence

Reflex Urinary Incontinence

Stress Urinary Incontinence

Total Urinary Incontinence

Urge Urinary Incontinence

Risk for Urge Urinary Incontinence

Disorganized Infant Behavior

Risk for Disorganized Infant Behavior

Readiness for Enhanced Organized Infant Behavior

Ineffective Infant Feeding Pattern

Risk for Infection

Risk for Injury

Risk for Perioperative-Positioning Injury

Decreased Intracranial Adaptive Capacity

Deficient Knowledge

Readiness for Enhanced Knowledge (Specify)

Risk for Loneliness

Impaired Memory

Impaired Bed Mobility

Impaired Physical Mobility

Impaired Wheelchair Mobility

Nausea

Unilateral Neglect

Noncompliance

Imbalanced Nutrition: Less than Body Requirements

Imbalanced Nutrition: More than Body Requirements

Readiness for Enhanced Nutrition

Risk for Imbalanced Nutrition: More than Body Requirements

Impaired Oral Mucous Membrane

Acute Pain

Chronic Pain

Readiness for Enhanced Parenting

Impaired Parenting

Risk for Impaired Parenting

Risk for Peripheral Neurovascular Dysfunction

Risk for Poisoning

Post-Trauma Syndrome

Risk for Post-Trauma Syndrome

Powerlessness

Risk for Powerlessness

Ineffective Protection

Rape-Trauma Syndrome

Rape-Trauma Syndrome: Compound Reaction

Rape-Trauma Syndrome: Silent Reaction

Impaired Religiosity

Readiness for Enhanced Religiosity

Risk for Impaired Religiosity

Relocation Stress Syndrome

Risk for Relocation Stress Syndrome

Ineffective Role Performance

Sedentary Life Style

Bathing/Hygiene Self-Care Deficit

Dressing/Grooming Self-Care Deficit

Feeding Self-Care Deficit

Toileting Self-Care Deficit

Readiness for Enhanced Self-Concept

Chronic Low Self-Esteem

Situational Low Self-Esteem

Risk for Situational Low Self-Esteem

Self-Mutilation

Risk for Self-Mutilation

Disturbed Sensory Perception (Specify: Visual, Auditory, Kinesthetic, Gustatory, Tactile, Olfactory)

Sexual Dysfunction

Ineffective Sexuality Patterns

Impaired Skin Integrity

Risk for Impaired Skin Integrity

Sleep Deprivation

Disturbed Sleep Pattern

Readiness for Enhanced Sleep

Impaired Social Interaction

Social Isolation

Chronic Sorrow

Spiritual Distress

Risk for Spiritual Distress

Readiness for Enhanced Spiritual Well-Being

Risk for Suffocation

Risk for Suicide

Delayed Surgical Recovery

Impaired Swallowing

Effective Therapeutic Regimen Management

Ineffective Therapeutic Regimen Management

Readiness for Enhanced Management of Therapeutic Regimen

Ineffective Community Therapeutic Regimen Management

Ineffective Family Therapeutic Regimen Management

Ineffective Thermoregulation

Disturbed Thought Processes

Impaired Tissue Integrity

Ineffective Tissue Perfusion (Specify Type: Renal, Cerebral, Cardiopulmonary, Gastrointestinal, Peripheral)

Impaired Transfer Ability

Risk for Trauma

Impaired **U**rinary Elimination

Readiness for Enhanced **U**rinary Elimination

Urinary Retention

Impaired Spontaneous **V**entilation

Dysfunctional **V**entilatory Weaning Response

Risk for Other-Directed **V**iolence

Risk for Self-Directed **V**iolence

Impaired **W**alking

Wandering

From Nursing Diagnosis: Definitions & Classification, 2005–2006, *by North American Nursing Diagnosis Association, 2005. Philadelphia: Author. Copyright 2005 by North American Nursing Diagnosis Association. Reprinted with Permission*

Appendix F: Abbreviations, Acronyms, and Symbols

AA	Alcoholics Anonymous
AA	arachidonic acid
AANA	American Association of Nurse Anesthetists
AAP	American Academy of Pediatrics
ABC	airway breathing circulation
ABG	arterial blood gas
ACE	angiotensin-converting enzyme
ACOG	American College of Obstetricians and Gynecologists
ACS	American Cancer Society
ACTG	AIDS Clinical Trial Group
ADH	antidiuretic hormone
ADOPE	age, diabetes, obesity, postterm, excessive
AFDC	Aid to Families with Dependent Children
AFP	alpha-fetoprotein
AFV	amniotic fluid volume
AGA	appropriate for gestational age
AHCPR	Agency for Health Care Policy and Research
AHNA	American Holistic Nurses Association
AHPA	American Herbal Products Association
AHRQ	Agency for Healthcare Research and Quality
AI	adequate intake
AICR	American Institute for Cancer Research
AIDS	acquired immunodeficiency syndrome
AMA	American Medical Association
ANA	American Nurses Association
ANAD	Anorexia Nervosa and Associated Disorders
ANDMCN	American Nursing Division of Maternal Child Nursing
ANRED	Anorexia Nervosa and Related Eating Disorders
ANS	autonomic nervous system

194

AOA	Administration on Aging
APIB	Assessment of Premature Infant Behavior
APN	advanced practice nurse
APS	Adult Protective Services
ARBD	Alcohol Related Birth Defects
AROM	artificial rupture of membranes
ART	assistive reproduction technology
AUB	abnormal uterine bleeding
AWHONN	Association of Women's Health, Obstetric, and Neonatal Nurses
AZT	zidovudine
β-hCG	β-human chorionic gonadotropin
BBT	basal body temperature
BINS	Bayley Infant Neurodevelopmental Screen
BMC	bone mineral content
BMD	bone mineral density
BMR	basal metabolic rate
BNE	Board of Nursing Examiners
BP	blood pressure
bpm	beats per minute
BPP	biophysical profile
BRP	bed rest bathroom privileges
BSE	breast self-examination
BUBBLE-HE	breasts, uterus, bladder, bowel, lochia, episiotomy, Homan's Sign, emotional status
BUN	blood urea nitrogen
Ca	calcium
CAM	complementary and alternative medicine
CBC	complete blood count
CCES	Council of Childbirth Education Specialists
CDC	Centers for Disease Control and Prevention
CDH	Congenital diaphragmatic hernia
CF	cystic fibrosis
C-H	crown-heel
CHARGE	coloboma, heart disease, choanal atresia, retardation (physical and mental), genital hypoplasia, ear anomalies
CHD	congenital heart defect
CHD	coronary heart disease
CHF	congestive heart failure
CHO	carbohydrate
CIMS	Coalition for Improved Maternity Services
CIS	Communities in Schools
cm	centimeter
CMV	cytomegalovirus
CNM	Certified Nurse Midwife
CNS	central nervous system

CO_2	carbon dioxide
COC	combined oral contraceptive
COPD	chronic obstructive pulmonary disease
CPAP	continuous positive airway pressure
CPD	cephalopelvic disproportion
CPR	cardiopulmonary resuscitation
CPS	Canadian Paediatric Society
C-R	crown-rump
CRNA	Certified Registered Nurse Anesthetist
CRS	congenital rubella syndrome
CSF	cerebrospinal fluid
CST	contraction stress test
CT	complementary therapy
CT	computerized tomography
CVD	cardiovascular disease
CVS	chorionic villus sampling
D & C	dilation and curettage
D & E	dilation and evacuation
DDH	developmental dysplasia of the hip
DDT	dichlorodiphenyltrichloroethane
DES	diethylstilbestrol
DFE	dietary folate equivalent
DHA	docosahexaenoic acid
DHHS	Department of Health and Human Services
DIC	disseminated intravascular coagulation
dL	deciliter
DMD	Duchenne muscular dystrophy
DMPA	depot medroxyprogesterone acetate
DMPA	Depo-Provera
DNA	deoxyribonucleic acid
DO	Doctor of Osteopathy
DRI	Dietary Reference Intake
DRV	daily reference value
DSHEA	Dietary Supplement Health and Education Act
DTR	deep tendon reflex
DUB	dysfunctional uterine bleeding
DV	daily value
EA	esophageal atresia
ECG	electrocardiogram
ECI	Early Childhood Intervention
ECMO	extracorporeal membrane oxygenation
EDB	expected date of birth
EDC	expected date of confinement
EDD	expected date of delivery
EDNP	energy-dense, nutrient-poor

EEG	electroencephalogram
EFM	electronic fetal monitoring
EFNEP	Expanded Food and Nutrition Education Program
EIP	early intervention program
ELISA	enzyme-linked immunosorbent assay
EMLA	eutectic mixture of local anesthetics
ER	estrogen receptors
ERT	estrogen replacement therapy
ESPGN	European Society of Pediatric Gastroenterology and Nutrition
ET	embryo transfer
FAE	fetal alcohol effects
FAS	fetal acoustic stimulation
FAS	Fetal Alcohol Syndrome
FCMC	family-centered maternity care
FDA	Food and Drug Administration
FFN	fetal fibronectin
FH	familial hypercholesterolemia
FHR	fetal heart rate
FHT	fetal heart tone
FMC	fetal movement counting
FOBT	fecal occult blood test
FOC	frontal-occipital-circumference
FPAL	full-term deliveries/preterm deliveries/abortions/living children
FSE	fetal scalp electrode
FSH	follicle-stimulating hormone
ftc	footcandle
g	gram
G6PD	glucose-6-phosphate dehydrogenase
GAO	General Accounting Office
GBS	group B *Streptococcus*
GCT	genetic counseling team
GFR	glomerular filtration rate
GI	gastrointestinal
GIFT	gamete intra-fallopian transfer
gm	gram
GNP	gross national product
GnRH	gonadotropin releasing hormone
H & H	hematocrit and hemoglobin
HbeAg	hepatitis B e antigen
HBIG	hepatitis B immune globulin
HBsAG	hepatitis B surface antigen
HC/AC	head-abdomen circumference
HCADA	Houston Council on Alcoholism and Drug Abuse
hCG	human chorionic gonadotropin
Hct	hematocrit

HDL	high-density lipoprotein
HDN	hemolytic disease of the newborn
HEENT	head, ears, eyes, nose, and throat
HELLP	hemolysis, elevated liver enzymes, low platelets
HexA	hexosaminidase
HFA	Healthy Families Alexandria
Hgb	hemoglobin
HGH	Human Growth Hormone
HGP	Human Genome Project
HGPRT	hypoxanthine-guanine phosphoribosyl-transferase
HHCC	Home Health Care Classification
HIV	human immunodeficiency virus
HMG	hydroxymethylglutaryl
HMO	health maintenance organization
HNC	Holistic nurse certification
HNC	Holistic Nurse Certified
hPL	human placental lactogen
HPV	human papillomavirus
HRT	hormone replacement therapy
HSV	herpes simplex virus
HT	Healing Touch
HTI	Healing Touch International
HTLV-1	human T-cell leukemia virus type 1
HVAF	Home Visiting for At-Risk Families
IBFAN	International Breastfeeding Association
ICEA	International Childbirth Education Association
ICH	intracranial hemorrhage
ICSI	intracytoplasmic sperm injection
ICU	intensive care unit
IDDM	insulin-dependent diabetes mellitus
IDM	infant of a diabetic mother
IF	intrinsic factor
IFSP	Individual Family Service Plan
IgA	immunoglobulin A
IgE	immunoglobulin E
IgG	Immunoglobulin G
IICP	increased intracranial pressure
ILCA	International Lactation Consultants Association
ILP	interstitial lymphocytic pneumonia
IM	intramuscular
IMR	infant mortality rate
in	inch
IOM	Institute of Medicine
IQ	intelligence quotient
ISONG	International Society of Nurses in Genetics

ITP	idiopathic thrombocytopenic purpura
IUD	intrauterine device
IUFD	intrauterine fetal demise
IUGR	intrauterine growth restriction
IUPC	intrauterine pressure catheter
IV	intravenous
IVF	in vitro fertilization
IVH	intraventricular hemorrhage
IWL	insensible water loss
JCAHO	Joint Commission on Accreditation of Healthcare Organizations
JOGNN	Journal of Obstetric, Gynecologic, and Neonatal Nursing
KC	kangaroo care
kg	kilogram
LAM	lactational amenorrhea method
lb	pound
LBW	low birth weight
LDL	low-density lipoprotein
LDR	labor, delivery, recovery
LDRP	labor, delivery, recovery, postpartum
LEEP	Loop Electrosurgical Excision Procedure
LGA	large for gestational age
LH	luteinizing hormone
LLI	LaLeche League International
LMA	left-mentum-anterior
LMP	last menstrual period
LMP	left-mentum-posterior
LMT	left-mentum-transverse
LOA	left-occiput-anterior
LOP	left-occiput-posterior
LOT	left-occiput-transverse
LSA	left-sacrum-anterior
LSP	left-sacrum-posterior
LST	left-sacrum-transverse
LTV	long-term variability
μg	microgram
m	meter
MAI	Maternal Attachment Inventory
MCV	mean corpuscular volume
Mg	magnesium
mg	milligram
MI	myocardial infarction
mL	milliliter
mmHg	millimeters of mercury
MNF	multiple neurofibromatosis
MPA/E2C	medroxy progesterone and estradiol cypionate

MPS	mucopolysaccharide accumulation
MRFIT	Multiple Risk Factor Intervention Trial
MRI	magnetic resonance imaging
MSAFP	maternal serum alpha-fetoprotein
MSDS	Material Safety Data Sheet
MVU	Montivideo Unit
NAACOG	Nurses Association of the American College of Obstetricians and Gynecologists
NANBH	non-A, non-B hepatitis
NANDA	North American Nursing Diagnosis Association
NANN	National Association of Neonatal Nurses
NAS	National Academies of Science
NBAS	Neonatal Behavioral Assessment Scale
NCAST	Nursing Child Assessment Satellite Training
NCCAM	National Center for Complementary and Alternative Medicine
NCEA	National Center for Elder Abuse
NCHPEG	National Coalition for Health Professional Education in Genetics
NCHS	National Center for Health Statistics
NCPAP	nasal continuous positive airway pressure
NCPCA	National Committee to Prevent Child Abuse
NE	niacin equivalent
NEC	necrotizing enterocolitis
NHANES	National Health and Nutrition Examination Society
NIC	Nursing Intervention Classification
NICU	neonatal intensive care unit
NIDCAP	Newborn Individualized Developmental Care Assessment Program
NIH	National Institutes of Health
NIHF	nonimmune hydrops fetalis
NIPS	Neonatal Infant Pain Scale
NLN	National League for Nursing
NMDS	nursing minimum data set
NRC	National Research Council
NSAID	nonsteroidal anti-inflammatory drug
NST	nonstress test
NTD	neural tube defect
NVP	nausea and vomiting of pregnancy
O_2	oxygen
OAM	Office of Alternative Medicine
OCA	oral contraceptive agents
OCP	oral contraceptive pill
OI	osteogenesis imperfecta
OMAR	Office of Medical Applications and Research
OMH	Office of Minority Health
ORWH	Office of Research on Women's Health

OSHA	Occupational Safety and Health Administration
OTC	over-the-counter
oz	ounce
P	phosphorus
PAI	Prenatal Attachment Inventory
PaO_2	partial pressure of oxygen
PAT	Pain Assessment Tool
PBB	polybromated biphenyl
PCA	patient-controlled analgesia
PCB	polychlorinated biphenyl
PCO_2	partial pressure of carbon dioxide
PCOS	polycystic ovary syndrome
PCP	*Pneumocystis carinii* pneumonia
PCR	polymerase chain reaction
PDA	patent ductus arteriosis
PDR	Physicians' Desk Reference
PEEP	positive and expiratory pressure
PEPI	postmenopausal estrogen/progestin interventions
PG	phosphatidylglycerol
PGE_2	prostaglandin E_2
PGIS	Perinatal Grief Intensity Scale
PHS	Public Health Service
PID	pelvic inflammatory disease
PIH	pregnancy-induced hypertension
PIPP	Premature Infant Pain Profile
PKU	phenylketonuria
PLISSIT	permission, limited information, specific suggestions, intensive therapy
PMI	point of maximum impulse
PMS	premenstrual syndrome
PNI	psychoneuroimmunology
PO_2	partial pressure of oxygen
POS	point of service
PPHN	persistent pulmonary hypertension of the newborn
PPO	preferred provider organization
PPROM	preterm premature rupture of membranes
PPT	partial prothrombin time
PROM	premature rupture of membranes
PT	prothrombin time
PTL	preterm labor
PTSD	Post-Traumatic Stress Disorder
PTT	partial thromboplastin time
PTU	propylthiouracil
PUBS	percutaneous umbilical blood sampling
PUPPP	pruritic urticarial papules and plaques of pregnancy

PVR	pulmonary vascular resistance
RBC	red blood cell
RD	registered dietitian
RDA	recommended daily allowance
RDI	Reference Daily Intake
RDS	respiratory distress syndrome
REEDA	redness, edema, ecchymosis, discharge, approximation
Rh	rhesus factor
RH_0GAM	Rh_o (D) immune globulin
RMA	right-mentum-anterior
RMP	right-mentum-posterior
RMT	right-mentum-transverse
RNA	ribonucleic acid
ROA	right-occiput-anterior
ROM	range of motion
ROM	rupture of membranes
ROP	retinopathy of prematurity
ROP	right-occiput-posterior
ROT	right-occiput-transverse
RSA	right-sacrum-anterior
RSP	right-sacrum-posterior
RST	right-sacrum-transverse
RUQ	right upper quadrant
SC disease	sickle cell-hemoglobin C disease
SCD	sickle-cell disease
SDA	specific dynamic action
SGA	small for gestational age
SIDS	sudden infant death syndrome
sIgA	secretory immunoglobulin A
SLE	systemic lupus erythematosus
SOAP	subjective, objective, assessment, plan
SQ	subcutaneous
SS disease	sickle cell disease
STD	sexually transmitted disease
STORCH	syphilis, toxoplasmosis, other infections, rubella, cytomegalovirus, herpes
STV	short term variability
SVE	sterile vaginal examination
TB	tuberculosis
TC	total cholesterol
TCM	traditional Chinese medicine
TEF	tracheoesophageal fistula
TENS	transcutaneous electrical nerve stimulation
THF	tetrahydrofolate
TNM	tumor, nodal involvement, and metastasis

TOLAC	trial of labor after cesarean
TORCH	toxoplasmosis, other (gonorrhea, syphilis, varicella, Parvovirus, HBV, and HIV), rubella, Cytomegalovirus, and herpes simplex virus
TPR	temperature, pulse, respirations
TRH	thyrotropin-releasing hormone
TSD	Tay-Sachs disease
TSH	thyroid-stimulating hormone
TT	Therapeutic Touch
TTN	transient tachypnea of the newborn
UAP	unlicensed assistive personnel
UC	uterine contraction
uE_3	unconjugated estrogen
UIL	upper intake level
UNAIDS	Joint United Nations Programme on HIV/AIDS
UNICEF	United Nations's Children's Fund
US	Ultrasonography
USDA	United States Department of Agriculture
USDA/FCS	United States Department of Agriculture, Food, and Consumer Service
USDHHS	United States Department of Health and Human Services
USFDA	United States Food and Drug Administration
USP	United States Pharmacopoeia
USPSTF	United States Preventive Services Task Force
UTI	urinary tract infection
VACTERL	vertebral, anal, congenital heart defect, tracheoesophageal atresia or fistula, renal anomalies, and limb deformities
VATER	vertebral, anal, tracheoesophageal atresia or fistula, and renal anomalies
VBAC	vaginal birth after cesarean
VDRL	Venereal Disease Research Laboratory
VLBW	very low birth weight
VNA	Visiting Nurse Association
VNS	Visiting Nurse Service
VPS	ventricular peritoneal shunt
VSD	ventricular septal defect
VZIG	varicella-zoster immune globulin
WABA	World Alliance for Breastfeeding Action
WBC	white blood cell
WHO	World Health Organization
WIC	Women, Infants, and Children
YRBSS	Youth Risk Behavior Surveillance System
ZDV	zidovudine

Appendix G: Preparation for NCLEX

The future belongs to those who believe in the beauty of their dreams.

(Eleanor Roosevelt)

A new graduate from an educational program that prepares registered nurses will take the NCLEX, the national nursing licensure examination prepared under the supervision of the National Council of State Boards of Nursing. NCLEX is taken after graduation and prior to practice as a registered nurse. The examination is given across the United States. Graduates submit their credentials to the state board of nursing in the state in which licensure is desired. Once the state board accepts the graduate's credentials, the graduate can schedule the examination. This examination ensures a basic level of safe registered nursing practice to the public. The examination follows a test plan formulated on four categories of client needs that registered nurses commonly encounter. The concepts of the nursing process, caring, communication, cultural awareness, documentation, self-care, and teaching/learning are integrated throughout the four major categories of client needs (Table G-1).

■ TOTAL NUMBER OF QUESTIONS ON NCLEX

Graduates may receive anywhere from 75 to 265 questions on the NCLEX examination during their testing session. Fifteen of the questions are questions that are being piloted to determine their validity for use in future NCLEX examinations. Students cannot determine whether they passed or failed the NCLEX examination from the number of questions they receive during their session. There is no time limit for each question, and the maximum time for the examination is 5 hours. A 10-minute break is mandatory after 2 hours of testing. An optional 10-minute break may be taken after another 90 minutes of testing.

204

TABLE G-1   NCLEX Test Plan: Client Needs

Client Needs Tested	Percent of Test Questions
Safe, effective care environment:	
Management of care	7-13%
Safety and infection control	5-11%
Physiologic integrity:	
Basic care and comfort	7-13%
Pharmacological and parenteral therapies	5-11%
Reduction of risk potential	12-18%
Physiological adaptation	12-18%
Psychosocial integrity:	
Coping and adaptation	5-11%
Psychosocial adaptation	5-11%
Health promotion and maintenance:	
Growth and development through the life span	7-13%
Prevention and early detection of disease	5-11%

Each test question has a test item and four possible answers. If the student answers the question correctly, a slightly more difficult item will follow, and the level of difficulty will increase with each item until the candidate misses an item. If the student misses an item, a slightly less difficult item will follow, and the level of difficulty will decrease with each item until the student has answered an item correctly. This process continues until the student has achieved a definite passing or definite failing score. The least number of questions a student can take to complete the exam is 75. Fifteen of these questions will be pilot questions, and they will not count toward the student's score. The other 60 questions will determine the student's score on the NCLEX.

■ RISK FACTORS FOR NCLEX PERFORMANCE

Several factors have been identified as being associated with performance on the NCLEX examination. Some of these factors are identified in Table G-2.

■ REVIEW BOOKS AND COURSES

In preparing to take the NCLEX, the new graduate may find it useful to review several of the many NCLEX review books on the market. These review books often include a review of nursing content, or sample test questions, or both. They frequently include computer software disks with test questions for review.The test questions may be arranged in the review book by clinical content area, or they may be presented in one or more comprehensive

206   Appendix G

TABLE G-2   Factors Associated with NCLEX Performance

- HESI Exit Exam
- Mosby Assesstest
- NLN Comprehensive Achievement test
- NLN achievement tests taken at end of each nursing course
- Verbal SAT score
- ACT score
- High school rank and GPA
- Undergraduate nursing program GPA

- GPA in science and nursing theory courses
- Competency in American English language
- Reasonable family responsibilities or demands
- Absence of emotional distress
- Critical thinking competency

examinations covering all areas of the NCLEX. Listings of these review books are available at *www.amazon.com*. It is helpful to use several of these books and computer software when reviewing for the NCLEX.

NCLEX review courses are also available. Brochures advertising these programs are often sent to schools and are available in many sites nationwide. The quality of these programs can vary, and students may want to ask former nursing graduates and faculty for recommendations.

■ THE NLN EXAMINATION AND THE HESI EXIT EXAM

Many nursing programs administer an examination to students at the completion of their nursing program. Two of these exams are the NLN Achievement test and the HESI Exit Exam. New graduates will want to review their performance on any of these exams because these results will help identify their weaknesses and help focus their review sessions.

Students who examine their feedback from the NLN examination or the HESI Exit Exam have important information that can help them focus their review for the NCLEX. A strategy for examining this feedback and organizing this review is outlined in the following section.

■ ORGANIZING YOUR REVIEW

In preparing for NCLEX, identify your strengths and weaknesses. If you have taken the NLN examination or the HESI Exit Exam, note any content strength and weakness areas. Additionally, note any nursing program course or clinical content areas in which you scored below a grade of B. Purchase one or more of the NCLEX review books. It is useful to review questions developed by different authors. Review content in the review books in any of your weak content areas.Take a comprehensive exam in the review book or on the computer software disk and analyze your performance. Try to answer as many questions correctly as you can. Be sure to actually practice taking the examinations. Do not just jump ahead to look at the section on correct answers and rationales before answering the questions if you want to improve your examination performance.

Next, once you have completed the comprehensive examination, review the answers and rationales for any weak content areas and take another comprehensive exam. Repeat this process until you are doing well in all clinical content areas and in all areas of the NCLEX examination plan.

Finally, do a general review of the top 10 patient diseases, medications, diagnostic tests, and nursing procedures in each major nursing content area, as well as defense mechanisms, communication tips, and growth and development. Practice visualization and relaxation techniques as needed. These strategies will assist you in conquering the three areas necessary for successful test taking—anxiety control, content review, and test question practice. Table G-3 will help organize your study.

TABLE G-3   Preparation for the NCLEX Test

Name: _____

Strengths: _____

Weak content areas identified on NLN examination or HESI Exit Exam:
_____
_____
_____

Weak content areas identified by yourself or others during formal nursing education pro-gram (include content areas in which you scored below a grade of B in class or any fac-tors from Table G-2):
_____
_____
_____

Weak content areas identified in any area of the NCLEX test plan, including the following:
    Safe, effective care environment

    Physiological integrity

    Psychosocial integrity

    Health promotion and maintenance

Continued

TABLE G-3   Continued

Weak content areas identified in any of the top 10 patient diagnoses in each of the following:
   Adult health

   Women's health

   Mental health nursing

   Children's health
   (Consider the 10 top medications, diagnostic tools and tests, treatments and procedures used for each of the ten diagnoses.)

Weak content areas identified in the following:
   Therapeutic communication tools

   Defense mechanisms

   Growth and development

   Other

■ WHEN TO STUDY

Identify your personal best time. Are you a day person? Are you a night person? Study when you are fresh. Arrange to study 1 or more hours daily. Use Table G-4 to organize your study if you have 1 month to go.

Students who use this technique should increase their confidence in their ability to do well on the NCLEX.

TABLE G-4   Organizing Your NCLEX Study

Note your weaknesses identified in Table G-3.

Take a comprehensive exam from one of the review books and analyze your performance. Then, depending on this test performance and the weaknesses identified in Table G-3, your schedule could look like the following:

Day 1:   Practice adult health test questions. Score the test, analyze your performance, and review test question rationales and content weaknesses.

Day 2:   Practice women's health test questions. Repeat above process.

Day 3:   Practice children's health test questions. Repeat above process.

Day 4:   Practice mental health test questions. Repeat above process.

Day 5:   Continue with other weak content areas. Continue this process until you are doing well in all areas of the test.

Glossary

A

ABO incompatibility Condition that occurs when the blood types of the mother and fetus do not match.

Accretion Growth in size, especially by addition or accumulation.

Acquaintance rape Sexual assault that occurs when a perpetrator with whom the victim has had a previous nonviolent relationship uses deceit and coercion to obtain sex.

Acquired disorder Condition resulting from environmental factors, rather than genetic circumstances.

Acupressure Application of pressure along certain meridians of the skin.

Acupuncture Insertion of needles into the skin along certain meridians.

Adolescence Period of life beginning with the appearance of secondary sex characteristics and ending with the cessation of growth, approximately 11 to 18 years of age; passage from childhood to maturity.

Adolescent pregnancy Pregnancy in girls, ages 11 to 19.

Adult maltreatment syndrome ICD-9 diagnostic code category for the adult who is abused.

Advanced reproductive age Women between ages 45 and 50 who are perimenopausal or postmenopausal.

Allantois Small diverticulum of the yolk sac.

Allele Alternative expressions of a gene at a given locus.

Allopathy Traditional or established medical or surgical procedures, both invasive and noninvasive, used in the diagnosis and treatment of mental or physical illnesses.

Alpha-fetoprotein (AFP) Protein produced by the developing fetus that can be used as a market for neural-tube defects (increased AFP) and Down syndrome (decreased AFP).

Alternative therapies Therapies used instead of conventional biomedicine.

Alveoli Secretory units of the mammary gland in which milk production takes place.

Amenorrhea The absence of menstruation for 3 or more months in women who have established menstrual cycles.

Amniocentesis Prenatal diagnostic procedure that consists of withdrawal of a small sample of amniotic fluid for genetic analysis of embryonic cells.

Amnion Inner membrane of the two fetal membranes; it forms the sac in which the fetus and the amniotic fluid are contained.

Amniotic fluid Fluid surrounding the developing fetus during pregnancy;

formed from maternal serum and fetal urine.

Amylophagia Ingestion of nonfood substances, such as laundry starch or cornstarch.

Analgesia Relief of pain.

Anencephalus Complete or partial absence of the cerebral hemispheres and the skull overlying the brain.

Anencephaly Fatal condition in which a baby is born with a severely underdeveloped brain and skull and dies shortly after birth.

Anesthesia Absence of sensation.

Anesthesiologist Physician who has completed a post-graduate residency in anesthesia.

Aneuploidy Abnormal chromosome pattern, in which the total number of chromosomes is not a multiple of the haploid number (n=23).

Anorexia nervosa Condition of self-starvation motivated by excessive concern with weight and an irrational fear of becoming fat.

Anovulatory Lack of ovulation.

Anovulatory cycle Menstrual cycle in which no ovum is discharged.

Antioxidant A substance that slows down the oxidation of hydrocarbons, oils, fats, etc. and thus helps to check deterioration.

Antiretroviral therapy Course of medications used to suppress HIV replication and viral load.

Areola Pigmented ring of tissue surrounding the nipple.

Asphyxia Interference with gas exchange, resulting in decreased oxygen delivery (hypoxemia), accumulation of carbon dioxide (hypercapnia), development of respiratory and metabolic acidosis, and inadequate perfusion of the tissues and major organs (ischemia).

Assault The intentional act of inflicting physical injury on another person.

Attachment Process of connecting with another human being over time.

Autonomy An individual's ability to hold a particular view, make choices, and undertake actions based on values and beliefs.

Autosome The 22 pairs of chromosomes that do not greatly influence sex determination at conception; excludes the sex chromosomes, X and Y.

Ayurvedic medicine Traditional medicine of India, meaning knowledge of life or science of longevity.

B

Ballottement Rebounding of the floating fetus against the examiner's fingers.

Barrier to service utilization Any deterrent either real or perceived, that presents or delays use of available health care.

Basal metabolism Energy used to support body functions while the body is at rest.

Behavioral medicine Branch of medicine that focuses on behavior, and the cognition, emotion, motivation and biobehavioral interactions.

Behavioral state Continuum of levels of consciousness, encompassing quiet sleep, drowsiness, wakeful attentiveness, and hyperalert, agitated, or crying states.

Beneficence The practice of doing good, which may include prevention of harm, removal of evil, or promotion of good.

Binge eating An eating disorder of periodic binge eating (several thousand calories) not normally followed by vomiting, the use of laxatives, or excessive exercise.

Bioavailability Rate at which a nutrient enters the bloodstream and is circulated to specific organs or tissues.

Biomedicine The scientific-based professional medicine that is taught in medical schools and is generally practiced in the United States and Canada.

Biophysical profile (BPP) Noninvasive, dynamic assessment of the fetus and the fetal environment.

Birth rate Number of births per 1,000 population.

Blastocyst Mammalian conceptus in the post-morula stage; consists of the trophoblast and an inner cell mass; develops into the embryo.

Blended family Family formed through remarriage.

Body mass index (BMI) Ratio that defines the relationship between height and weight. BMI is calculated by the formula: BMI = weight (kg)/height (m^2) × 100, or weight (lb) × 700/height (in^2).

Botanicals All parts of plants that have medicinal value: roots, rhizomes, leaves, stems, and flowers.

Brachial palsy Paralysis of the muscles involving the upper extremity; occurs as a result of a prolonged and difficult labor followed by a traumatic delivery.

Braxton-Hicks contractions Intermittent painless contractions of the uterus, observed throughout pregnancy; also known as false labor.

Bulimia nervosa Condition characterized by bingeing, or excessive consumption of calories over a short period of time, and purging by self-induced vomiting, use of laxatives or diuretics or both, excessive exercise or periods of severe caloric restriction.

C

Calorie Amount of energy needed to raise the temperature of 1/kg of water (about 4 cups) 1°C.

Calorimetry Measurement of the quantity of heat; used for measuring the energy produced by food when oxidized in the body.

Capacitation Process by which the spermatozoon (sperm) is capable of penetrating the ovum.

Carcinoma in situ Cancer that involves only the cells of the organ in which it began and has not spread to any other tissue.

Carotenoids Pigments in fruits and vegetables, which include alphacarotene, beta-carotene, lycopene, lutein, and many other compounds.

Case management, care coordination Process of coordinating care and services to assure that clients receive appropriate care and services in a timely manner.

Categorical imperative Supreme rule that governs actions.

Certified Registered Nurse Anesthetist (CRNA) Advanced practice nurse, graduated from an accredited program of nurse anesthesia education who has passed the National Certification Examination.

Cervical cancer Neoplasm of the uterine cervix.

Cervical infection Inflammation of the cervix caused by a microorganism or foreign body.

Chadwick's sign Dark blue or purple coloration of vaginal mucous membranes during pregnancy.

Chi A concept in Oriental medicine that refers to the subtle material or energy that influences physiologic function and maintains the health and vitality of the individual.

Chi gong The oriental practice of "working the chi", or exercises to maintain health and vitality.

Child abuse Physical or mental injury, sexual abuse, exploitation, negligent treatment, or maltreatment of a child.

Chloasma Brownish pigmentation of the face, commonly called "mask of pregnancy."

Choanal atresia A bony or membranous separation between the nose and the pharynx.

Chorion Outermost portion of the fetal membrane; composed of trophoblast and mesoderm lining; develops villi and becomes vascularized; forms the fetal portion of the placenta.

Chorionic villi Vascular protrusions along the chorion.

Chorionic villus sampling (CVS) Procedure to obtain fetal cells in the first trimester of the developing pregnancy.

Chromosome Filament-like nuclear structure, consisting of chromatin, which stores genetic information as base sequences in DNA and whose number is constant in each species.

Civil law Rule protecting individuals, which punishes wrongs against the individual.

Clastogen Agent capable of producing chromosome breakage.

Cleft lip Congenital fissure or elongated opening of the lip.

Cleft palate Congenital fissure in the palate.

Clubfoot (talipes eqiunovarus) Congenital deformity in which portions of the foot and ankle are twisted out of normal position.

Code Definition of professional obligations and responsibilities, expected of practitioners by society.

Cognitive development Age-related development of intellectual reasoning and perception.

Cohabitation Couple living together without entering into marriage.

Colostrum A yellowish, protein-rich fluid, secreted from the breast during pregnancy and for 3 to 4 days following delivery.

Communal family Group of individuals, couples, or families living together and jointly carrying out family functions.

Complementary therapies Therapies used in addition *to* or as an *adjunct* to biomedicine for the promotion of health and well being.

Congenital disorder Anomaly present at birth; results from genetic or prenatal environmental factors, or both.

Congenital heart defect A structural abnormality or defect of the heart that is present at birth.

Contraction stress test (CST) Evaluation of uterine contractions for the purpose of assessing fetal response.

Corona radiata Layer of cells surrounding the zona pellucida of the ovum.

Corpus luteum Yellow glandular mass in the ovary formed by an ovarian follicle that has matured and discharged its ovum.

Cost-benefit analysis Process of measuring the cost of doing something against the outcome in monetary terms.

Cost-effectiveness analysis Process of comparing the cost of doing something and measuring the outcomes in non-monetary terms.

Cotyledons Subdivisions along the uterine surface of the placenta.

Couvade Physical symptoms experienced by an expectant father during pregnancy; also the ritualistic behaviors he performs during labor and birth.

Criminal law Rule that addresses public concerns and punishes the wrongs that threaten a group or society.

Crisis Situation in which the balance in individual or family life is disrupted and new coping strategies must be developed.

Critical thinking Formal and structured type of reasoning that is used in nursing as the foundation for sound clinical judgement.

Cultural competence Process of integrating cultural awareness in the delivery of culturally appropriate clinical care.

Cultural competence continuum - Progressive description of the ability of an individual or institution to respond to the individual, culturally specific needs of people.

Culture An individual's way of looking at life, encompassing the person's feelings, beliefs, attitudes, and practices in dealing with family, community, and society.

Cytogenetics The study of chromosomes, with special focus on chromosome abnormalities.

Cytotrophoblast Inner layer of the trophoblast; also referred to as Langhan's layer.

D

Daily Reference Values (DRVs) Standards for daily intake of total fat, saturated fat, cholesterol, total carbohydrate, dietary fiber, and protein.

Date rape Assault between a dating couple without consent of one of the participants.

Decidua Term applied to the endometrium during pregnancy.

Decidua basalis Portion on which the implanted ovum rests.

Decidua capsularis Portion directly overlaying the implanted ovum.

Decidua vera Decidua exclusive of the area occupied by the implanted ovum.

Deletion Loss of chromosomal material.

Deontology Form of ethical reasoning that focuses on duty; right actions are those that fulfill duty.

Dermatome The area of the body innervated through a specific spinal nerve.

Desire phase First phase of human sexual response in which a person develops a motivation or intention to be sexual.

Developmental care Infant care protocol designed to promote optimal physical, cognitive, and emotional development in the first weeks or months of life.

Developmental crisis Adjustment of an individual to new stages of development.

Developmental dysplasia of the hip (DDH) Malformation of the hip involving varying degrees of deformity, ranging from subluxation to complete dislocation, that may be present at birth.

Developmental tasks Competencies in psychosocial development related to identity formation, sexual identity, vocational identity, and autonomy and independence.

Diaphragmatic hernia Condition in which the diaphragm fails to close during the seventh or eighth week, allowing the abdominal organs to be displaced into the left chest.

Dietary Guidelines for Americans Guidance on diet and health for the general population with practical recommendations that meet nutritional requirements, promote health, support an active lifestyle, and reduce the risk of chronic disease.

Dilemma Choice between two equally unsatisfactory alternatives.

Diploid Cell that contains two copies of each chromosome; the diploid number (2n) in humans is 46.

Disease prevention Activities taken to prevent the onset of a disease or disorder.

Doctrine of the golden mean Virtues at the midpoint between extremes of less desirable characteristics.

Dominant Allele that is phenotypically expressed in single copy (heterozygote), as well as in double copy (homozygote).

Doppler blood studies Measurement of blood flow velocity and direction in major fetal and uterine structures; also known as umbilical vessel velocimetry.

Dosha A term used in Ayurvedic medicine referring to metabolic types of people.

Ductus arteriosus Fetal shunt that connects the pulmonary artery to the descending aorta.

Ductus venosus Fetal shunt passing through the liver that connects the umbilical vein to the inferior vena cava.

Due care Legal and ethical standards of performance by which nursing professionals are expected to abide.

Dyads Group of two people.

Dysfunctional uterine bleeding (DUB) Any significant deviation from the usual menstrual pattern; also known as abnormal uterine bleeding (AUB).

Dysmenorrhea Painful menses or cramping with menstruation.

Dyspareunia Painful sexual intercourse.

E

ECMO Extracorporeal membrane oxygenation, a method of cardiopulmonary bypass therapy.

Ecologic environment Combined social context in which a family resides.

Elderly primigravida Woman over age 35 who is pregnant for the first time.

Embryo Period of human development from the second week until the eighth week after fertilization; period characterized by cell differentiation and hyperplasic growth.

Embryo transfer (ET) Transfer of an externally fertilized egg in embryonic stage by transcervical or other methods.

Empowering A therapeutic approach that encourages the family to actively participate in the solution to their problems, and acknowledge that capacity.

Empowerment Process of assisting clients to care for themselves.

Enablement Process of assisting clients in locating needed services and resources.

Enabling The approach to interventions that allow competencies to develop in the client.

Encephalocele Herniation of the brain and meninges through a skull defect.

Endometrial cancer Malignant neoplasm of the uterine lining.

Endometriosis Chronic disorder caused by implantation of endometrial tissue outside the uterus.

Endometrium Cellular lining of the uterus that is shed monthly at the time of menses.

En-face positionings Face-to-face positioning between parent and newborn.

Engorgement The process of swelling of the breast tissue due to vascular congestion following delivery and preceding lactation.

Engrossment Process characterized by intense parental interest in the newborn.

Enhancement Process of building on a client's existing strengths in order to increase capacity for problem solving and self-care.

Epidural A technique used to produce analgesia or anesthesia of the lower body by placing opioid and/or local anesthetic within the epidural space, which then diffuses into the nerve roots as they exit the dura.

Epispadias Condition in which the urethral meatus is located on the dorsal surface of the penis.

Erythroblastosis fetalis Vast destruction of fetal red blood cells by maternal antibodies, resulting in fetal anemia.

Esophageal atresia Condition in which the esophagus ends in a blind pouch or narrows into a thin cord and is not connected to the stomach.

Estrogen Female sex hormone produced primarily by the ovary and stored in fat cells.

Estrogen deficiency vulvovaginitis - Vulvo vaginal burning related to estrogen decline.

Ethnic of care Perspective that recognizes the personal concerns and vulnerabilities of clients in health and illness.

Ethics Rules and principles that can be used for resolving ethical dilemmas.

Ethnic group Community of people who share the same cultural and social beliefs, which have been passed from one generation to another.

Euploid Cell (and, by extension, an individual) whose chromosome number is a multiple of 23.

Evidence-based practice Systematic approach to finding, appraising and judiciously using research results as a basis for clinical decisions.

Excitement phase Phase of the human sexual response in which physical and emotional changes take place in the person to increase interest in intercourse.

Exstrophy of the bladder Anomaly in which the anterior wall of the bladder and lower portion of the abdominal wall are absent, causing the bladder to lie open and exposed on the lower abdomen.

Extended family Family which includes generations beyond the parents and their children, such as grandparents or aunts and uncles; or two or more nuclear families together.

Extrauterine life Life outside of the uterus following birth.

F

Facial palsy Paralysis of one side of the face.

False discharge Fluid appearing on the nipple or areolar surface that is not secreted by breast tissue.

Family Group of adults and children linked by biological, kinship, or social bonds.

Family boundaries The demarcations between individuals within a family and between the family and the rest of society.

Family dynamics Concept from psychology that refers to the patterns in the interrelationships within the family.

Family structure Configuration of the family unit, including who is in the family and their relationship to each other.

Femicide Homicide of women.

Fertility rate Number of births per 1,000 women of ages 15 to 44.

Fertilization Process by which the male's sperm unites with the female's ovum.

Fetal circulation The pathway of blood circulation in the fetus.

Fetal fibronectin (fFN) testing Screening procedure for the prediction of preterm labor.

Fetal movement counting (FMC) Daily maternal assessment of fetal activity by counting the number of fetal movements within a specified time period.

Fetal tissue sampling Direct biopsy of fetal tissue.

Fibroadenoma Painless solid breast mass or tumor.

Fibrocystic changes Hormonal age-related changes, most commonly involving cyst formation and thickening of breast tissue.

Fibroid tumor Benign tumor arising in the myometrium, which can protrude into the uterine cavity, bulge through the outer uterine layer, or grow within the myometrium.

Fidelity Quality of being faithful.

Fimbriae Fine hair-like structures.

Follicle stimulating hormone (FSH) Hormone produced by the anterior pituitary whose function is to stimulate the ovary to prepare a mature ovum for release.

Follicular phase Phase of the ovarian cycle in which a follicle becomes mature and prepared for ovulation.

Follow-up services Health care services provided following hospital discharge.

Food Guide Pyramid Translation of the Dietary Guidelines for Americans into practical eating portions and, if foods are chosen carefully, they also meet the Recommended Daily Allowances (RDA) and Dietary Reference Intakes (DRI).

Foramen ovale An opening in the septum between the right and the left atria of the fetal heart.

Foremilk Thin watery breastmilk secreted at the beginning of a feeding.

G

Galactopoiesis The maintenance of established lactation.

Galactorrhea White discharge from the nipples.

Gamete Mature reproductive cell; spermatozoon or ovum.

Gametogenesis Series of mitotic and meiotic divisions that occurs in the gonads and leads to the production of gametes; in males, spermatogenesis, and in females, oogenesis.

Gastroschisis Abdominal wall defect to the right of the umbilicus through which the abdominal organs herniate.

Gene Segment of nucleic acid that contains genetic information necessary to control a certain function, such as the synthesis of a polypeptide (structural gene); also referred to as a site, or locus, on a chromosome.

General anesthesia Loss of sensation from the entire body secondary to loss of consciousness produced by intravenous and/or inhalation anesthetic agents.

Genetic counseling Process by which genetic information is given to clients and their families.

Genetic disorder Inherited defect that is transmitted from generation to generation.

Genotype Genetic constitution of an individual at any given locus.

Geophagia Ingestion of nonfood substances, such as dirt or clay.

Germ cells Precursors of the ova.

Goals Broad statements of a desired outcome.

Gonadal Pertaining to the ovaries in the female and the testes in the male.

Gonadotropin-releasing hormone (Gm-RH) Neurohormone released by the hypothalamus that acts on the pituitary to stimulate the release of follicle-stimulating hormone, luteinizing hormone, thyroid stimulating hormone, and prolactin.

Goodell's sign Marked softening of the cervix in early pregnancy.

Graafian follicle   Fully mature ovum and surrounding elements just before ovulation.

H

Habituation   A newborn's ability to alter response to a repeated stimulus by decreasing and finally eliminating the response after repetitions of the stimulus.

Haploid   Cell that contains one copy of each chromosome; the haploid number (n) in humans is 23.

Harm   Interference with the mental or physical well-being of others.

Healing   To make whole and incorporates physical, psychological, social, spiritual and environmental health and may or may not include cure.

Health care informatics   Integration of computer science, information science and various health care professionals involved in collecting, processing and managing data.

Health promotion   Process, action, program, or endeavor to obtain the goal of complete physical, mental, and social well-being.

Hegar's sign   Softening of the isthmus of the uterus in pregnancy.

Heme iron   A type of iron from animal sources, which constitutes about half of the iron available from animal sources.

Hemizygous   Condition in which an allele is present in a single copy.

Hemochromatosis   Rare genetic defect in iron metabolism, in which excess iron is deposited in the tissues, causing abnormal skin pigmentation, hepatic cirrhosis and decreased carbohydrate tolerance, which eventually ends in multiple-organ failure.

Hemosiderosis   Iron storage disorder that results in iron toxicity.

Herbs   Leafy plants that do not have woody stems.

Heterozygote   Individual who has two different alleles at a given locus on a pair of homologous chromosomes.

Hindmilk   Thicker, high-fat breastmilk, secreted at the end of a feeding.

Holism   Philosophy of integration of body, mind and spirit within a dynamic environment.

Home care   Provision of technical, psychological, and other therapeutic support in the client's home environment rather than in an institution.

Home care nursing   Delivery of nursing care in the home environment.

Home visit   Visit occurring in the family's place of residence or in any such facility where a family may be housed, such as a homeless shelter, group home, church or halfway house.

Homologous   Refers to chromosomes with matching genes, or to those genes individually.

Homozygote   Individual who has a pair of identical alleles at a given locus.

Human chorionic gonadotropin (hCG)   Hormone secreted by the corpus luteum of the ovary after conception.

Human immunodeficiency virus (HIV) and acquired immunodeficiency syndrome (AIDS)   Retrovirus that causes progressive and severe impairment of the body's natural immunologic function, resulting in serious opportunistic infections, various cancers, and eventual death (AIDS).

Human placental lactogen (hPL)   Produced by the syncytiotrophoblast cell as early as 3 weeks after ovulation and is detectable in the maternal serum at 4 weeks after fertilization.

Hydrocele   Collection of serous fluid in the scrotum.

Hydrocephaly Condition that results from an excess accumulation of cerebrospinal fluid (CSF) in the ventricles of the brain, caused by an imbalance between CSF production and absorption.

Hydrops fetalis Severe form of fetal hemolytic disease; severe anemia results in hypoxia, cardiac decompensation, and hepatosplenomegaly.

Hyperbilirubinemia Elevated level of bilirubin in the blood.

Hyperemesis gravidarum Severe vomiting during pregnancy.

Hypocalcemia A low level of calcium in the blood; (less than 7 mg/dL).

Hypochromic anemia Anemia characterized by red blood cells lacking in color.

Hypoglycemia A less than normal amount of glucose in the blood; in the newborn, a plasma glucose level of less than 40 mg/dL.

Hypophyseal-pituitary-ovarian axis Transport mechanism of gonadotropin-releasing hormone from the hypothalamus that stimulates the release of gonadotropins from the anterior pituitary that, in turn, causes stimulation of the ovaries to release estrogen and progesterone.

Hypospadias Congenital anomaly in which the urethral meatus is located on the ventral surface of the glans penis instead of at the end.

Hypothalamic-pituitary-gonadal axis Triad of the hypothalamus, pituitary, and ovaries that must function in synchrony for conception to occur.

Hypothermia Rectal or axillary temperature below 97.0°F.

Hypovolemia Decreased circulating blood volume.

I

Imperforate anus A group of anatomic anomalies of the rectum and anus.

Implantation Embedding of the fertilized ovum into the endometrium.

Impotence Inability of the male to achieve or maintain an erection.

Incest Sexual relations between blood relatives or surrogate family members.

Infant of a diabetic mother (IDM) Infant born to a mother who has diabetes mellitus.

Infertility Diminished or absent ability to produce an offspring despite regular unprotected intercourse for 1 year.

Informed consent Information regarding treatment procedures are given to clients, and their consent is secured.

Insoluble fiber Fiber that resists absorption into the body.

Integrated medicine Provision of health care services combining both biomedical and complementary medicine.

Interdisciplinary teams Health care that is delivered by individuals from various disciplines that share responsibility, authority and decision making.

Intracranial hemorrhage Collection of blood within the cranium.

Intrathecal A technique used to produce analgesia of the lower body by placing a small amount of opioid drug into the cerebral spinal fluid.

Invasive breast cancer Cancer that has extended beyond the local epithelium and has the potential to spread from the breast to other parts of the body.

Invasive cancer Cancer that has spread or infiltrated beyond the original site or organ.

J

Jaundice Accumulation of bilirubin; produces a yellow discoloration of the newborn's skin, mucous membranes, and sclera.

Justice Division of benefits and burdens in society.

K

Kangaroo care Skin to skin contact between mother and infant.

Karyotype Chromosome constitution of an individual, represented by a laboratory-made display in which chromosomes are arranged by size and centromere position.

Kernicterus Excess accumulation of unbound, unconjugated bilirubin, deposited in brain tissues, especially the basal ganglia.

L

La Leche League International organization that promotes breastfeeding.

Lactation consultant Specially trained health care provider whose primary focus is providing breastfeeding assistance to help new mothers in establishing breastfeeding.

Lactational discharge Any secretory discharge occurring as a physiologic response to the normal hormonal stimulation of pregnancy, postpartum, or after weaning.

Lactogenesis The process of milk production 2-5 days postpartum.

Langhan's layer Inner layer of the trophoblast; also referred to as the cytotrophoblast.

Lanugo Downy hair that is present on the fetus between the 20th week and birth.

Latching-on Proper attachment of the infant to the breast for feeding.

Law Rules governing human behavior that represent the minimum standard of morality.

Let-down reflex Milk ejection from the breast triggered by nipple stimulation or emotional response to the infant.

Letting-go phase Final phase of maternal adjustment characterized by role attainment and relationship adjustment.

Leydig cells Interstitial tissue cells of the testes that produce testosterone.

Liability Accountability for professional conduct according to standards that have been set.

Libido Conscious or unconscious sexual desire.

Life expectancy Average number of years for which a group of individuals of the same age are expected to live.

Linea nigra Dark line of pigmentation that extends from the symphysis pubis to the umbilicus, at midline on the abdomen during pregnancy.

Local anesthetic Class of drugs that produce reversible blockade of electrical impulses along nerve fiber.

Local infiltration anesthesia Loss of sensation in a small area due to blockade of neural impulses as a result of infiltration of tissue with an anesthetic drug such as lidocaine.

Localized breast cancer Cancer that has not metastasized, is usually less than 2 cm in size, is considered noninvasive beyond the breast, and has the best outcome.

Luteal phase Phase of the ovarian cycle after ovulation when the corpus luteum secretes hormones to prepare the uterine endometrium for implantation until the placenta matures and assumes the function of providing nutrients for the embryo.

Luteinizing hormone (LH) Anterior pituitary hormone whose surge occurs immediately before ovulation and is responsible for release of the ovum.

M

Macro-environment Elements that define the caregiving milieu, that is, conditions that define the surrounding space in which caregiving occurs.

Macronutrients   Any of the chemical elements, such as carbon, required in relatively large quantities for growth.

Macrosomatia   Birth weight above the 90th percentile for gestational age, or a birth weight of more than 4 kg (8 lb, 12.8 oz).

Magnetic resonance imaging (MRI)   Noninvasive diagnostic tool that provides high-resolution cross-sectional images of fluid-filled soft tissues.

Malpractice   Negligence involving the actions of professionals.

Managed care   Health care plans with a selected list of providers and institutions from which the recipient is entitled to receive health care that is reimbursed by the insurer.

Mastectomy   Excision (removal) of the breast.

Mastitis   Infection in the breast, usually confined to a milk duct, characterized by influenza-like symptoms and redness and tenderness in the infected breast.

Material principles of justice   Guidelines that can be used to justify the distribution of benefits.

Maternal sensitization   Process by which the maternal immunologic system forms antibodies against fetal blood cells.

Maternal serum–α-fetoprotein (MS-AFP) testing   Screen of maternal blood for the presence and volume of alpha-feto protein (AFP).

Maternal-infant bonding   The forming of an emotional attachment between mother and newborn.

Mature milk   Breast milk that contains 10% solids for energy and growth.

Meconium   Initial stool developed in the fetus; it is viscid, sticky, dark in color, sterile, and odorless.

Meconium staining   Staining of the newborn's skin and nails; results from fetal passage of stool in utero.

Medical model   Biomedical approach to health care that is oriented to treating specific diagnosis and focused on physical problems.

Meiosis   Process by which germ cells divide and decrease their chromosomal number by half.

Menarch   Establishment or beginning of the menstrual function.

Menarche   Initiation of the first menses.

Meningocele   Spinal cord defect in which an external sac that protrudes through the defect and contains meninges and cerebrospinal fluid.

Menopause   Natural or surgically imposed cessation of menses.

Menses   Monthly bleeding from the lining of the uterus.

Menstrual phase   Phase of the menstrual cycle when a woman experiences vaginal bleeding.

Meridian   In Oriental medicine, the channels or pathways in the body through which Chi travels.

Mesenchyme   Meshwork of embryonic connective tissue that forms the connective tissue of the body, blood vessels, and lymph vessels.

Metastatic breast cancer   Breast cancer that is found in parts of the body in addition to the breasts.

Microcephaly   A small brain in a normally well-formed head.

Microcytic anemia   Anemia characterized by red blood cells of small size.

Micro-environment   Elements that are specifically related to the individual infant's environment or care experiences.

Micronutrients   Any of the chemical elements, such as iron, required in minute quantities for growth.

Mitosis Process in which body cells duplicate themselves and then separate into two new daughter cells.

Mittelschmerz Abdominal pain occurring at the time of ovulation.

Monosomy Aneuploid condition of having a chromosome represented by a single copy in a somatic cell, i.e., the absence of a chromosome from a given pair.

Morbidity rate Ratio of the number of cases of a disease or a condition to a given population.

Mortality rate Ratio of the number of deaths in various categories to a given population.

Morula Solid mass of cells formed by cleavage of a fertilized ovum.

Mosaicism Condition that results in an individual (mosaic) with two or more genetically different cell populations.

Moxibustion In Oriental medicine, the burning of herbs near the skin in order to affect movement of Chi.

Multifactorial Resulting from interactions between genetic and environmental factors.

Mutation Abrupt genetic alteration in an individual, which is transmitted to the offspring.

Myelomeningocele Spinal cord defect in which part of the spinal cord is herniated into the external sac, which contains meninges, cerebrospinal fluid, and neural tissue.

N

Neglect Withholding of essential components of daily living, such as food, clothing, medications, and shelter.

Negligence Unintentional wrong caused by failure to act as a reasonable person would under similar circumstances.

Neurohormonal Pertaining to hormones formed by neurosecretory cells and liberated by nerve impulses.

Neutral thermal environment A set of environmental conditions created to maintain the normal body temperature; minimizes oxygen consumption and caloric expenditure.

Nipple discharge Fluid produced by and accumulating within a secretory unit of the breast, exiting through the nipple.

Nondisjunction Failure of homologous chromosomes, or chromatids, to separate properly during anaphase meiosis I and II, or mitosis, resulting in daughter cells with unequal chromosome numbers; meiotic nondisjunction may result in gametes with abnormal chromosome number, which upon fertilization may produce aneuploidy; mitotic nondisjunction that occurs in a developing embryo may result in mosaicism.

Nonheme iron Dietary iron from foods other than meats, in which the iron is not bound in the hemoglobin molecule; comprises half of the iron found in animal sources and all of the iron found in plant sources, including grains and cereals.

Nonmaleficence Acting to prevent harm to others.

Nonstress test (NST) Evaluation of fetal heart rate in response to an increase in either spontaneous or stimulated fetal activity.

Nuchal cord Umbilical cord encircling the fetal neck.

Nuclear family Family composed of two generations, parents and their children.

Nutrition Facts Food Label Labeling on processed packaged foods that lists credible health and nutrient content claims, standardized serving sizes, and the Percent Daily Values (DV), based on a 2000-calorie diet.

O

Obesity Body weight of 20% or more over ideal body weight.

Objectives Specific short-term achievements expected to result in the accomplishment of the goal. These are generally written in specific measurable outcomes.

Omphalocele Defect covered by a peritoneal sac at the base of the umbilicus, into which portions of the abdominal organs herniate.

Opioid A type of drug which binds to opioid receptors and produces a degree of analgesia. Morphine and Demerol are two drugs of this type.

Organogenesis Development of organs.

Orgasmic phase Phase of the human sexual response after the plateau phase in which immense sexual tension is released.

Osteoporosis Progressive bone loss, increased bone fragility, and increased risk for bone fractures, which occurs in postmenopausal women.

Ovarian cancer Malignant neoplasm of the ovary.

Ovulation Release of a mature ovum in preparation for conception.

Oxytocin Hormone produced by the posterior pituitary that stimulates uterine contractions and the release of milk from the mammary glands.

P

Pagophagia Ingestion of nonfood substances, such as ice and ice frost.

Parenteral Administration of drug via intramuscular or intravenous routes.

Paternalism Interference in the liberty of a person, in which the interference is justified by promoting the well-being of that individual.

Pathologic discharge Results from pathologic conditions affecting the hypothalamic-pituitary axis, prolactin levels, or breast diseases that affect both breasts.

Pathologic jaundice Jaundice of the newborn caused by the excessive breakdown of red blood cells as a result of hematologic incompatibility.

Pedigree (genogram) Diagram that describes family relationships and gender, disease status, and other relevant information about a family.

Pelvic inflammatory disease (PID) Inflammation of the uterus, fallopian tubes, or ovaries caused by ascent of vaginal flora or bacteria.

Pelvic relaxation The loss of muscle support of the pelvic organs.

Percutaneous umbilical blood sampling (PUBS) Evaluation technique that provides direct access to the fetal circulation and involves direct aspiration of fetal blood.

Perimenopause Time period before the cessation of menses.

Perpetrator Person accused of a criminal offense.

Persistent pulmonary hypertension A condition caused by a sustained elevation in pulmonary vascular resistance after birth, preventing the transition to the normal extrauterine circulatory pattern.

Phenotype Any observable or measurable expression of gene function.

Phototherapy Ultraviolet light used for treatment of jaundice in the newborn.

Physiologic anemia of pregnancy - Disproportionate increase of the plasma volume compared with the red blood cell volume, resulting in a lower-than-normal hemoglobin level and hematocrit during pregnancy.

Physiologic discharge Result of physiologic conditions affecting all breast tissue equally, involving secretory tissue in each breast and resulting in milky white or multicolored fluid.

Physiologic jaundice Benign form of jaundice that usually occurs after the third day of life and is caused by the normal break-down of superfluous red blood cells.

Phytochemicals Plant-based chemicals.

Phytotherapy The therapeutic use of plants, often referring to herbal remedies.

Pica Psychobehavioral disorder that manifests as persistent ingestion of substances having little or no nutritional value or craving of unnatural articles as food during pregnancy.

Plateau phase Phase of human sexual response occurring just before orgasm.

Plumbism Ingestion of nonfood substances, such as lead paint flakes.

Polycystic ovary syndrome Endocrine disorder characterized by long-term anovulation and an excess of androgens circulating in the blood; characterized by formation of cysts in the ovaries, a process related to the failure of the ovary to release an ovum.

Polycythemia Increased number of red blood cells.

Polygenic Referring to a trait whose phenotypic expression results from the cooperation of various genes.

Postnatal circulation The normal extrauterine circulatory pattern of blood flow through the heart, lungs, and body.

Prana A term used in Ayurvedic medicine referring to vital energy.

Precocious Developing maturity very early or rapidly.

Premature ovarian failure Failure of ovarian estrogen production and ovulation after menarche and before age 40, in which the woman experiences the symptoms of menapause.

Premenstrual syndrome Cyclic cluster of behavioral, emotional, and physical symptoms, which occur during the luteal phase of the menstrual cycle and are of sufficient severity to interrupt normal activity.

Preterm An infant born at less than 38 weeks' gestation.

Prima facie A conditional duty that can be overridden by a more stringent duty.

Primary amenorrhea Absence of menarche until age 16 or absence of the development of secondary sex characteristics and menarche until age 14.

Primary apnea A self-limited condition characterized by absence of respiration; occurs in the early stage of asphyxia.

Primary dysmenorrhea Painful menses from uterine causes but without pelvic pathology; usually occurs within 3 years of onset of menstrual cycling.

Proactive Development of capacity to deal with stressors prior to a crises.

Proband Clinically identified person who displays the characteristics or features of a disease; also referred to as index case, or propositus (fem, proposita).

Progesterone Antiestrogenic hormone produced by the corpus luteum of the ovary that assists in maintenance of pregnancy through implantation.

Prolactin Hormone from the pituitary gland that triggers milk production in response to tactile stimulation of the breast.

Proliferative phase Phase of the menstrual cycle in which the endometrium becomes prepared for implantation.

Prostaglandins Class of hormones found in many tissues that affects vasodilation, constriction, and uterine smooth muscle.

Pseudomenstruation Pinkish-white mucoid vaginal discharge noted shortly after birth owing to maternal transfer of estrogen.

Puberty Period in which the secondary sex characteristics begin to develop and the capability of sexual reproduction is attained; onset of the process of physical maturity.

Pudendal block A technique using local anesthesia to block transmission through the pudendal nerves.

Pulmonary vascular resistance Resistance in the pulmonary vascular bed against which the right ventricle must eject blood.

Q

Quickening First fetal movement, felt by the mother; usually noticed at about 18 to 20 weeks' gestation.

R

Race A group of people defined by similar physical features, such as skin color, facial features, and texture of body hair.

Rape Nonconsensual sexual penetration of another by force or threat of force.

Recessive Allele whose phenotypic expression occurs in homozygous or hemizygous conditions.

Recommended Dietary Allowances (RDA) Average daily nutrient intake levels recommended for healthy Americans.

Reconstituted family Family formed through remarriage.

Reducing agent Any substance that reduces another substance, or brings about reduction, and is itself oxidized in the process.

Reference Daily Intakes (RDIs) Standard that addresses the vitamin and mineral content of foods.

Refractory period Period of time after orgasm when the human is incapable of further sexual activity.

Regional anesthesia Loss of sensation from a large area of the body due to blockade of neural impulses.

Relactation Reinstitution of lactation after it has been discontinued.

Renal solute load The sum of solutes that must be excreted by the kidneys.

Resolution phase Phase of human sexual response when the physiologic changes in the body that occur as a result of sexual activity return to normal.

Resuscitation Basic emergency procedure used for life support, consisting of airway management, positive pressure ventilation, chest compressions, medication, and thermal support.

Rh incompatibility (isoimmunization) Hemolytic disease caused by the incompatibility of Rh factors in maternal and fetal blood.

Risk assessment Process of examining the risk factors that may place an individual at risk for disease.

Role attainment Completing the developmental tasks of a new social role.

Role mastery Successful attainment of developmental tasks.

Role transition Process of adopting new behaviors to accomplish change and developmental tasks.

Rooting reflex Normal response of the newborn to move toward whatever touches the area around the mouth.

S

Screening A test or examination to detect the most characteristic sign or signs of a disorder or disease that may require further investigation.

Secondary amenorrhea Absence of menses for at least 6 months or for three cycles, after previously experiencing menstrual cycles.

Secondary apnea An abnormal condition that occurs in the late stages of asphyxia in which respiration is absent and does not resume spontaneously without resuscitation.

Secondary dysmenorrhea Painful menses accompanied by a pathologic process.

Secretory phase Phase of the menstrual cycle that occurs after ovulation and before menstruation.

Seminiferous tubules Tubules that carry semen from the testes.

Sepsis Systemic bacterial, viral, or parasitic infection that invades the bloodstream.

Serial monogamy Practice of having one sexual partner at a time but several partners during a lifetime.

Seroconversion Conversion of the blood serum from negative to positive for any infecting agent.

Sexual dysfunction Related to a disorder of one of the phases of human sexual response.

Sexual maturation Establishment of menstruation and ovulation in females and the development of spermatogenesis in males.

Situational crisis Event or situation that occurs in a personal or a family life, which requires the adaptation or acquisition of new coping mechanisms.

Sleep-wake cycle Stages of newborn sleep pattern.

Social assets Assets or benefits to ones health that are related to one's social position and socioeconomic status.

Soluble fiber Fiber that binds bile acids and coats the intestines, thus inhibiting absorption.

Somite One of the paired segments along the neural tube of the embryo.

Spermatogenesis Entire process of development and maturation of sperm cells.

Spermatozoa Male gamete or sex cell.

Spermatozoon Mature male germ cell (sperm); spermatozoa (plural).

Spina bifida Congenital defect in which the spinal canal does not close and protrudes from the back.

Spinnbarkeit Stringy elastic character of cervical mucus at time of ovulation.

Stalking "A course of conduct directed at a specific person that involves repeated visual or physical proximity, nonconsensual communication, violence toward property, verbal, written or implied threats, or a combination thereof" (Tjaden & Thoennes, 1998, p. 2).

Standards of care Documents developed by members of a profession to establish a mutually adopted level of practice.

STORCH An acronym used to describe a titer for syphilis, toxoplasmosis, other, rubella, cytomegalovirus, and herpes.

Stranger rape Nonconsensual sexual experience between a victim and assailant who are strangers.

Stress incontinence Involuntary discharge of urine with a cough, sneeze, or laughter owing to the loss of muscular support at the neck of the urethra.

Stressor Illness, that may result in change.

Striae gravidarum Pinkish or darkened streaks, resulting from stretching of the skin during pregnancy that occurs predominantly on the breasts and abdomen.

Subarachnoid hemorrhage Collection of blood in the subarachnoid space of the brain.

Supine hypotension   Condition of reduced blood flow to the right atrium when the pregnant woman lies in a supine position.

Surfactant   Complete lipoprotein that reduces the surface tension of pulmonary fluids, allowing the exchange of gases in the alveoli of the lungs.

Syncytiotrophoblast   Outer layer of the trophoblast.

Systemic vascular resistance   Resistance against which the left ventricle must eject its stroke volume with each heart beat.

T

Taking-hold phase   Second phase of maternal adjustment, characterized by an increased readiness to be involved with the newborn.

Taking-in phase   Initial, early period of maternal adjustment, characterized by basic maternal needs for food, care, and comfort.

Tanner Stages   Five stages of female and male physiologic development.

Teratogen   Environmental substance that can cause physical defects in the developing embryo and fetus.

Testosterone   Most potent naturally occurring androgen (male) hormone that is made in the testes, ovary, and adrenal cortex.

Thelarche   Beginning of the development of the breasts at puberty, with prominence of glandular tissue behind the nipples. The first sign of puberty.

Thermoregulation   The control of heat production and heat loss, specifically the maintenance of body temperature through physiologic mechanisms activated by the hypothalamus.

Tort   Civil wrong that may be caused either intentionally or unintentionally.

Tracheoesophageal fistula   Condition in which the trachea and esophagus are abnormally connected.

Transient tachypnea of the newborn   Mild, self-limited respiratory disorder, characterized by an increased respiratory rate and mild cyanosis and though to be related to delayed resorption of fetal lung fluid.

Transitional milk   Milk produced at the end of colostrum production and immediately before mature milk comes in the breast.

Translocation   Misplacement of genetic material from one chromosome to another.

Trisomy   Aneuploid condition caused by the presence of an extra chromosome, which is added to a given chromosome pair and results in a total number of 47 chromosomes per cell; Down syndrome is the most common human autosomal trisomy.

Trophoblast cells   Peripheral cells of the blastocyst that attach the fertilized ovum to the uterine wall and develop into the placenta and membranes.

U

Ultrasonography   Use of high-frequency ($>20,000$ Hz) sound waves to detect differences in tissue density and to visualize outlines of structures within the body.

Universalizability   Rule used to guide actions that could be followed in all other similar situations.

Upper intake level (UL)   Maximum level of daily nutrient intake.

Urge incontinence   Inability to postpone urination for more than a few minutes once the need to urinate is sensed. The bladder is unable to empty normally and becomes distended, which results in an uncontrolled loss of urine.

Utilitarianism   Type of ethical thinking focusing on the consequences of actions; actions are right if they bring about the best possible outcomes and the least bad effects for the greatest number of persons.

V

Vaginal infection   Inflammation of the vagina caused by a microorganism or foreign body.

Vaginismus   Painful spasms of the muscles of the introitus that prevent penetration.

Varicocele   Abnormal blood vessel in the scrotum.

Vegan   Vegetarian who consumes no animal products.

Veracity   Truthfulness.

Vertical transmission   Transmission of HIV by the mother to the fetus or neonate during pregnancy, delivery, and postnatally, during breastfeeding.

Virtue   Character trait that is valued.

Virtue ethics   The way in which personal characteristics of the moral agent or person guide moral action.

Vitalism   A term used in 19th Century Europe and America referring to a type of vital energy or life force.

W

Weaning   Process of discontinuing breastfeeding and accustoming an infant to another feeding method.

Wet nurse   Woman who breastfeeds for pay infants who are not her own.

Wharton's jelly   Soft, jelly-like substance of the umbilical cord.

Wife rape   Forced sexual experience with a common-law or legally married spouse.

Z

Zona pellucida   Transparent, noncellular layer surrounding the ovum.

Zygote   Cell resulting from the union of the ovum and spermatozoon.

Code Legend

NP	**Phases of the Nursing Process**
As	Assessment
An	Analysis
Pl	Planning
Im	Implementation
Ev	Evaluation

CN	**Client Need**
Sa	Safe Effective Care Environment
Sa/1	Management of Care
Sa/2	Safety and Infection Control
He/3	Health Promotion and Maintenance
Ps/4	Psychosocial Integrity
Ph	Physiological Integrity
Ph/5	Basic Care and Comfort
Ph/6	Pharmacological and Parenteral Therapies
Ph/7	Reduction of Risk Potential
Ph/8	Physiological Adaptation

CL	**Cognitive Level**
K	Knowledge
Co	Comprehension
Ap	Application
An	Analysis

SA	**Subject Area**
1	Medical-Surgical
2	Psychiatric and Mental Health
3	Maternity and Women's Health
4	Pediatric
5	Pharmacologic
6	Gerontologic
7	Community Health
8	Legal and Ethical Issues

228

Practice Test 1

THE ANTEPARTAL PERIOD - COMPREHENSIVE EXAM

1. At the first prenatal visit, the client reports the first day of her last menstrual cycle to be October 16. Based on Naegele's rule, the nurse determines the estimated date of confinement for the client is

   1. July 16 of the next year.

   2. August 16 of the next year.

   3. August 23 of the next year.

   4. July 23 of the next year.

2. During an eight-week prenatal visit, a client makes statements that lead the nurse to believe the client has mixed emotions about the pregnancy. Understanding the developmental tasks of pregnancy, the nurse assesses that the client is working through which task of pregnancy?

   1. Role transition

   2. Fetal embodiment

   3. Fetal distinction

   4. Pregnancy validation

3. A pregnant client has called to say she counted seven fetal movements while doing her daily fetal movement count for one hour. The nurse appropriately responds in which of the following manners?

   1. Gather more information about the client's activity and nutrition for the day

   2. Educate the client that babies often sleep for extended periods and inquire if this is the first time decreased fetal movement has been noticed

   3. Instruct the client to come in and have the decreased fetal movement evaluated

   4. Educate the client that seven fetal movements in one hour is reassuring

229

4. A pregnant client asks for more information about her screening prenatal ultrasound. Before responding, the nurse considers which of the following aspects of the screening ultrasounds?

    1. The screening prenatal ultrasound is done to look at the major organ systems for anomalies

    2. The screening ultrasound uses sound waves undetected by the human ear

    3. The screening ultrasound can be either transvaginally or transabdominally

    4. The screening ultrasound requires a small amount of radiation, which is considered safe for the fetus

5. The nurse assesses a pregnant client who began having severe abdominal pain. The client's clinical manifestations also include a hard, boardlike abdomen, hypotension, and tachycardia. The nurse calls for help and evaluates fetal heart tones suspecting

    1. an ongoing spontaneous abortion.

    2. placental abruption.

    3. placenta previa.

    4. a gallbladder attack.

6. Following amniocentesis for fetal lung maturity, the nurse implements which of the following interventions for the pregnant client?

    1. Vital signs and Doppler fetal heart rate

    2. Teach the client clinical manifestations of complications to report in the first 15 minutes

    3. Escort the client out of the building in a wheelchair

    4. Electronic fetal monitoring for a minimum of 30 minutes

7. The pregnant client is concerned because she is one week past her due date. The nurse responds based on knowledge of gestation. Which is the appropriate understanding of gestation? Term pregnancy is

    1. from the beginning of the 38th week until the end of the 42nd week.

    2. from the beginning of the 39th week until the 40th week.

    3. 36 weeks until 38 weeks.

    4. from the beginning of the 40th week until the end of the 40th week.

8. The nurse returns a call to a pregnant client who asks about her diagnosis of preterm labor. Based on an understanding of the condition, the nurse appropriately responds as follows.

    1. "You will deliver this baby early."

    2. "You have been having cervical dilation without contractions and you must stay on bed rest to slow the process."

3. "The contractions have been changing your cervix and it is too early before you reach term."

4. "Cervical dilation and effacement before your 20th week in this pregnancy is labor that is starting too soon and is called preterm labor."

9. A pregnant client is admitted to the hospital for an incomplete abortion. Which statement illustrates correct understanding of the nurse's teaching?

   1. "I will have to take iron when I go home."
   2. "I will not need RhoGam since my pregnancy didn't last."
   3. "I will need a D and C."
   4. "I will need surgery since the pregnancy was in my tube."

10. A client with gestational trophoblastic disease has asked about the need for contraception. The nurse's response is based on the understanding of follow-up care for this condition as follows.

    1. Once the disease is treated, the client's contraception plans have no influence on the client's wellness
    2. The client should be encouraged to use contraception for the next year
    3. The client is to be discouraged from using hormonal-only contraception, to not aid in the growth of further gestational trophoblastic disease
    4. The client should avoid progesterone-only contraception

11. A hospitalized pregnant client who is currently collecting a 24-hour urine informs the nurse that one void was missed. The nurse's intervention is based on the knowledge of the diagnostic procedure. Which intervention is appropriate?

    1. No intervention is required
    2. Ask the client to estimate the amount of the void that was missed and inform the lab when the urine is sent
    3. Inform the lab that one void was missed so the final report will include that disclaimer
    4. Discard the collected urine and begin the test over

12. During a contraction stress test (CST), a client demonstrates one fetal heart rate (FHR) acceleration for 15 seconds that was 15 beats above the baseline. No FHR decelerations were noted after uterine contractions. The nurse records the results as

    1. nonreactive, negative CST.
    2. nonreactive, positive CST.

3. reactive, negative CST.

4. reactive, positive CST.

13. A client pregnant at 35 weeks of gestation has phoned with the concern of leaking vaginal fluid. Which of the following is a consideration before responding to the client, based on an understanding of rupture of membranes in the preterm pregnancy? The client will need to

1. report to the hospital when the uterine contractions are five minutes apart.

2. report to the hospital immediately.

3. be placed on home bed rest.

4. keep her prenatal appointment tomorrow.

14. A pregnant client reports abstaining from drinking alcohol for one month, but she was overwhelmed with stress and began drinking again last week. The best response from the nurse is

1. "A month is better than nothing."

2. "Quitting for a month is great and must have been difficult."

3. "Unfortunately, your baby is still at risk from your previous drinking."

4. "Can you quit again?"

15. A pregnant client with a cervical cerclage in place has been determined to be in labor. Which statement evidences understanding of the nurse's teaching?

1. "The cerclage will prevent me from delivering."

2. "Once preterm labor begins, it cannot be stopped."

3. "I will receive indomethacin now that I am in labor."

4. "The cerclage will need to be removed."

16. The nurse recognizes which client is at risk for isoimmunization?

1. Rh-negative

2. Rh-positive

3. Both Rh-negative and -positive

4. Neither Rh-negative or -positive

17. Which client statement demonstrates the need for more nursing education about diabetes mellitus and pregnancy?

1. "Keeping my blood sugar under control is very important while my baby's body is forming."

2. "I will follow the diet prescribed."

3. "I will check my blood sugar at home three times a day."

4. "I have a higher risk of needing a cesarean section."

18. A pregnant client receives terbutaline (Brethaire) for preterm labor. The nurse should monitor the client for which of the following adverse reactions?

Select all that apply:

[   ] **1.** Transient hypotension

[   ] **2.** Constipation

[   ] **3.** Tachycardia

[   ] **4.** Diplopia

[   ] **5.** Cough

[   ] **6.** Heartburn

19. A client presents with the diagnosis of ectopic pregnancy. The nurse recognizes the priority nursing intervention is to

1. monitor the vital signs.

2. obtain a surgical consent.

3. allow the client and her family to grieve for the lost pregnancy.

4. ask the client about her blood type.

20. The client reports to the nurse that her fetus has been diagnosed with Turner's syndrome. The nurse understands this is a fetus with

1. XXY chromosomes.

2. XYY chromosomes.

3. XO chromosomes.

4. YO chromosomes.

21. After being hospitalized for pregnancy-induced hypertension (PIH), the client asks the nurse why the baby is in danger from her high blood pressure. The nurse responds based on which of the following?

1. The fetus's blood pressure will also be elevated

2. The placental perfusion is at risk

3. The client's headache will prevent her from taking in adequate nutrition

4. The client's hypertension early in pregnancy has already damaged the fetus

22. The nurse uses Nitrazine paper to test the vaginal fluid from a pregnant client who feels the membranes have ruptured. What should the nurse expect from the test if the membranes have ruptured?

1. Nitrazine paper should not change color

2. Nitrazine paper will be bright yellow

3. Nitrazine paper will turn a dark green

4. Nitrazine paper will turn blue

23. A pregnant client undergoing electronic fetal monitoring evidences a fetal heart rate of 190. The nurse interprets this as
    1. fetal tachycardia.
    2. normal.
    3. maternal tachycardia.
    4. normal variability.

24. During a prenatal appointment, the nurse evaluates the chart and notes that the 41-year-old client is at increased risk for delivering a child with what chromosomal abnormality?
    1. Down syndrome (trisomy 21)
    2. Cystic fibrosis
    3. Turner's syndrome
    4. Hemophilia

25. Which of the following should the nurse include in the plan of care for a client who is pregnant, has diabetes mellitus, and is taking insulin?
    1. Discontinue the insulin
    2. Decrease the dose of insulin
    3. Administer the same dose of insulin
    4. Increase the dose of insulin

26. The registered nurse is preparing the clinical assignments for a maternity unit. Which of the following nursing tasks should the nurse delegate to a licensed practical nurse?
    1. Assess a client for Braxton-Hicks contractions
    2. Provide the care for a client in pre-eclampsia
    3. Walk a client in her 37th week of gestation
    4. Instruct a client on the clinical manifestations of placenta previa

ANSWERS AND RATIONALES

1. 4. Naegele's rule is to count back three months from the first day of the last menstrual cycle and then add one year and seven days.
   NP = As
   CN = He/3
   CL = An
   SA = 3

2. 4. Initial ambivalence about the pregnancy is common in pregnancy validation. Role transitions include preparing to separate from the fetus,

anxiety about labor and delivery, exhibiting "nesting" behaviors, and feeling ready for the pregnancy to end. The woman in fetal embodiment encompasses the fetus into the body image. In fetal distinction, the woman conceptualizes the fetus as a separate individual.

NP = As
CN = He/3
CL = Ap
SA = 3

3. 3. A reassuring fetal movement count is ten movements in one hour and decreased fetal movement is an indication for further investigation. The client should be instructed to come in for an evaluation. A fetus may not be active if the mother has not eaten and the mother may have had so much activity that she failed to notice true fetal movements. Regardless, these possibilities do not negate the appropriate action to evaluate further simply on the client's report of decreased fetal movement.

NP = An
CN = He/3
CL = An
SA = 3

4. 2. The screening ultrasound uses sound waves, not radiation, and it is a transabdominal view of gross fetal features. A targeted or selective ultrasound views all organ systems for anomalies.

NP = An
CN = Ph/7
CL = Ap
SA = 3

5. 2. The hallmark clinical manifestations of placental abruption include severe abdominal pain with or without notable vaginal bleeding as the growing hematoma creates pressure inside the somewhat fixed uterine cavity. Hypotension and tachycardia result from maternal blood loss.

NP = Ev
CN = He/3
CL = An
SA = 3

6. 4. The fetal well-being must be evaluated for 30 minutes following amniocentesis. Electronic fetal monitoring provides more complete data than using a Doppler. The client should not leave right away.

NP = Im
CN = He/3
CL = Ap
SA = 3

7. 1. Term gestation is from the beginning of the 38th week of gestation to the end of the 42nd week.
NP = An
CN = He/3
CL = Ap
SA = 3

8. 4. Progressive cervical changes (dilation and effacement) between the 20th and the 37th week in the presence of regular uterine contractions are preterm labor.
NP = An
CN = He/3
CL = Ap
SA = 3

9. 3. An incomplete abortion is vaginal bleeding and cramping resulting in expulsion of part of the products of conception; the remaining tissue must be removed.
NP = An
CN = He/3
CL = Ap
SA = 3

10. 2. The client with gestational trophoblastic disease (hydatiform mole) is at risk of developing choriocarcinoma or malignant trophoblastic disease, and should avoid pregnancy for the next year in the event that chemotherapy is indicated. The type of contraception is not a factor. Also, regular follow-up in the next year is important for early detection of cancer.
NP = An
CN = He/3
CL = An
SA = 3

11. 4. The 24-hour urine results are not valid if even one void is missed. The urine must be discarded and the test will need to begin again.
NP = Im
CN = Ph/7
CL = Ap
SA = 3

12. 1. A contraction stress test must have a minimum of two FHR accelerations 15 beats over the baseline and lasting for 15 seconds to be reactive. The question also describes a negative CST, which is no FHR deceleration after contractions.
NP = An
CN = Ph/7

CL = An
SA = 3

13. 2. The client with preterm premature rupture of membranes will need to be hospitalized immediately to be observed for complications, which are life threatening for the client and fetus, and to begin IV antibiotic prophylaxis.
NP = An
CN = He/3
CL = An
SA = 3

14. 2. Telling a client that quitting for a month is great and must have been difficult acknowledges the client's efforts and does not judge the behavior.
NP = An
CN = He/3
CL = An
SA = 3

15. 4. The cerclage is a surgical procedure that sutures the cervix in the management of an incompetent cervix. The cervical cerclage will need to be removed for labor. The client is at risk for uterine or cervical rupture if labor continues with a cervical cerclage.
NP = Ev
CN = He/3
CL = Ap
SA = 3

16. 1. The client with Rh-negative is at risk for isoimmunization.
NP = As
CN = Ph/7
CL = An
SA = 3

17. 3. A client who is pregnant and has diabetes mellitus will need to check fasting blood sugar levels three times a day.
NP = Ev
CN = He/3
CL = Ap
SA = 3

18. 3, 5, 6. Adverse reactions to terbutaline (Brethaire), a sympathomimetic drug, include tachycardia, palpitations, nervousness or drowsiness, tremors, headache, pulmonary edema, cardiac arrhythmia, hyperglycemia, cough, and heartburn.
NP = As
CN = Ph/6

CL = Ap
SA = 5

19. 1. Vital signs are monitored for signs of hemodynamic instability, which could herald the rupture of the ectopic pregnancy and make the situation emergent.
NP = Im
CN = Sa/1
CL = An
SA = 3

20. 3. Turner's syndrome is a female with only one X chromosome.
NP = An
CN = He/3
CL = Co
SA = 3

21. 2. The placental blood flow is at risk from the vasoconstriction that is present in PIH. The condition can progress to pre-eclampsia and maternal seizures with eclampsia, which further compromises fetal blood flow.
NP = An
CN = He/3
CL = An
SA = 3

22. 4. Nitrazine paper will turn blue from the alkaline pH of amniotic fluid.
NP = Ev
CN = Ph/7
CL = Ap
SA = 3

23. 1. Normal fetal heart rate is 110 to 160.
NP = Ev
CN = Ph/7
CL = Ap
SA = 3

24. 1. The risk for Down syndrome increases each year after age 35.
NP = As
CN = He/3
CL = Ap
SA = 3

25. 4. Oral hypoglycemic medications are contraindicated in pregnancy and will be discontinued by the client who is pregnant. This client should be managed on insulin if a drug is necessary. More insulin is required as the pregnancy continues.
NP = Pl
CN = Ph/6

CL = Ap
SA = 5

26. 3. Assessing a client for Braxton-Hicks contractions, providing the care of a client in pre-eclampsia, and instructing a client on the clinical manifestations of placenta previa are tasks that require the skills of the registered nurse. A licensed practical nurse may walk a client who is pregnant.
NP = Pl
CN = Sa/1
CL = An
SA = 8

THE INTRAPARTAL PERIOD - COMPREHENSIVE EXAM

1. When a client who is pre-eclamptic complains of epigastric pain and nausea, which of the following disorders should the nurse consider as the priority explanation for causing these clinical manifestations?
    1. Ischemic changes in the liver
    2. Appendicitis
    3. Gastritis
    4. Peptic ulcer

2. A client who is pre-eclamptic is experiencing shortness of breath and chest pain. It is a priority for the nurse to notify the physician of which of the following suspected disorders?
    1. Myocardial infarction
    2. Pulmonary edema
    3. Pneumonia
    4. Bronchitis

3. After reviewing the laboratory reports on a client who is pregnant, the nurse should report which of the following?
    1. Hemoglobin of 14 g/dl
    2. Serum glucose of 88 mg/dl
    3. Hematocrit of 45%
    4. Platelet count of 50,000

4. Which of the following of Leopold's maneuvers should the nurse use to determine if the presenting part is engaged and the attitude of the head is in a cephalic presentation?
    1. First maneuver
    2. Second maneuver

3. Third maneuver

4. Fourth maneuver

5. The nurse should monitor for the potential complication of disseminated intravascular coagulation (DIC) when providing care to which of the following clients?

   1. A client who has a placenta previa

   2. A client who has abruptio placentae

   3. A client who is experiencing preterm labor

   4. A client who has had a rupture of the membranes

6. The nurse should administer what type of insulin and by what route to a client who has type 1 diabetes during labor? _____

7. The nurse should evaluate the fetal monitor tracing for which of the following for a client who develops hypotension?

   1. Late decelerations

   2. Early decelerations

   3. Variable decelerations

   4. Accelerations

8. Based on an understanding of nonsteroidal anti-inflammatories and their effect on the pregnant client, the nurse should understand that indomethacin (Indocin) may cause which of the following?

   1. Premature closure of the fetal ductus arteriosus

   2. Fetal tachycardia

   3. Fetal bradycardia

   4. Improvement of maternal asthma

9. When assessing a client in labor for admission, which question is a priority for the nurse to ask prior to performing a digital vaginal examination?

   1. "When did your contractions begin?"

   2. "How frequent are your contractions now?"

   3. "Have you had any vaginal bleeding during your pregnancy?"

   4. "Which pregnancy is this for you?"

10. The nurse is providing care to four clients in the labor and delivery unit. Which client should the nurse provide continuous electronic fetal monitoring?

    1. A client at 38 weeks of gestation in false labor

    2. A client who has had an uncomplicated pregnancy, in latent phase of stage 1

    3. A client at 25 weeks of gestation in premature labor

    4. A client who is gravida 2 para 1 who has had an uncomplicated pregnancy and is dilated 5 cm

11. After assessing the medical records of four clients admitted, which of the clients does the nurse prioritize as being at greatest risk of having a high-risk birth?

    1. A client who is 24 weeks pregnant and is having Braxton-Hicks contractions

    2. A sensitized Rh-negative client who is 24 weeks pregnant and has an Rh-positive fetus

    3. A client who is 16 weeks pregnant and frequently travels by airplane

    4. A client who has an Rh antibody titer of 1.0 and is 28 weeks pregnant

12. The nurse is performing an admission assessment on a client in early labor at 40 weeks of gestation and evaluates the normal fundal height to be

    1. 38 cm.

    2. 43 cm.

    3. 40 cm.

    4. 35 cm.

13. After performing Leopold's maneuvers on a client admitted and in labor, the nurse should prepare the client for a vaginal delivery after determining the fetus is in which of the following positions?

    1. Transverse lie

    2. Longitudinal, cephalic lie, vertex presentation

    3. Oblique lie

    4. Longitudinal, cephalic lie, face presentation

14. After performing a vaginal examination, Leopold's maneuvers, and evaluating the findings to be plus 3, longitudinal, cephalic, and fetal vertex, the nurse should document which of the following findings in the blank labeled presentation?

    1. Plus 3

    2. Oblique

    3. Cephalic

    4. Fetal vertex

15. The nurse caring for a client who is 5 cm dilated should follow the protocol for care of the client in

    1. latent phase, first stage of labor.

    2. transition, first stage of labor.

3. second stage of labor.

4. active phase, first stage of labor.

16. Which of the following clinical manifestations are priority for the nurse to report on a woman in the second stage of labor?
Select all that apply:

[   ] 1. Rigid, tender uterus

[   ] 2. Maternal urge to push

[   ] 3. Involuntary bearing down efforts

[   ] 4. Severe abdominal pain

[   ] 5. Bulging of the perineum

[   ] 6. Bright red bleeding

17. It is a priority for the nurse caring for a newly delivered mother to monitor the fundal height, fundal tone, lochia, and vital signs of a client who has a uterus that is boggy and fails to contract for which of the following?

1. Disseminated intravascular coagulation

2. Fever

3. Postpartum hemorrhage

4. Hematoma

18. A client at 38 weeks of gestation complains of pain in the "pubic bone" when walking. The nurse informs the client that this is laxity of the symphysis pubis due to which of the following hormones?

1. Progesterone

2. Estrogen

3. Relaxin

4. Melantropin

19. The nurse is caring for a mother whose fetus has died in utero. The mother is crying when the nurse enters the room. Which of the following is the appropriate response or action by the nurse?

1. "It may not feel like it, but it is better to happen now instead of after you have seen and held the child."

2. "It is God's way of telling you that the fetus was deformed in some way."

3. After placing a hand on the client's shoulder state, "I'm so sorry for your loss."

4. Provide the client with privacy and limit interactions with the client to providing care

ANSWERS AND RATIONALES

1. 1. While nausea and epigastric pain may be associated with appendicitis, gastritis, and peptic ulcer, they usually reflect ischemic liver changes in the pre-eclamptic client.
NP = An
CN = Ph/7
CL = An
SA = 3

2. 2. One of the manifestations of "third-spacing" of fluid in pre-eclampsia is pulmonary edema. While dyspnea and chest pain may occur in myocardial infarction, pneumonia, or bronchitis, these clinical manifestations are caused by pulmonary edema in pre-eclampsia.
NP = An
CN = Ph/7
CL = An
SA = 3

3. 4. A hemoglobin of 14 g/dl, serum glucose of 88 mg/dl, and hematocrit of 45% are all within normal limits. The platelet count is abnormal. Platelets do not normally change during pregnancy; thus, the platelet count of 50,000 is abnormal and should be reported to the physician promptly. A decrease in the platelet count (normal is 150,000 to 450,000) to 50,000 should indicate to the nurse a coagulation problem and pre-eclampsia.
NP = An
CN = Ph/7
CL = An
SA = 3

4. 3. Leopold's maneuver, or abdominal palpation, refers to the method of abdominal palpation used to determine fetal presentation and position. The third Leopold's maneuver is used to determine if the presenting part is engaged and the head is in cephalic presentation.
NP = Im
CN = He/3
CL = Ap
SA = 3

5. 2. The clot breakdown products (fibrin degradation products) produced in abruptio placentae are potent anticoagulants that may produce disseminated intravascular coagulation.
NP = As
CN = Ph/7
CL = An
SA = 3

6. **Infusion of regular insulin along with an IV glucose infusion by infusion pump.** IV insulin drip allows titration for control of blood glucose. Long-acting insulin should be avoided during labor.
   NP = Im
   CN = Ph/6
   CL = Ap
   SA = 5

7. 1. If hypotension interferes with uterine blood flow, uteroplacental insufficiency and late decelerations result.
   NP = Ev
   CN = He/3
   CL = An
   SA = 3

8. 1. Maintenance of the ductus arteriosus in the fetus requires prostaglandin E. Indomethacin (Indocin), like other NSAIDs, inhibits prostaglandin synthesis. Thus, it may cause premature closure of the ductus. Inhibition of prostaglandin synthesis can worsen maternal asthma. It has no direct effect on fetal heart rate.
   NP = An
   CN = Ph/6
   CL = An
   SA = 3

9. 3. If a client has current or prior vaginal bleeding, the nurse should not perform a digital vaginal examination.
   NP = As
   CN = Ph/7
   CL = Ap
   SA = 3

10. 3. The client in premature labor is at high risk and requires continuous fetal monitoring. A client who is at 38 weeks of gestation in false labor and clients in uncomplicated pregnancies are not at high risk, and intermittent monitoring may be appropriate.
    NP = Pl
    CN = Ph/7
    CL = An
    SA = 3

11. 2. Immunization or sensitization results when fetal blood enters the circulation of the mother, causing antibodies to be formed in the mother's blood. These formed antibodies cross the placenta and attack the fetal blood. As a result, there is a hemolysis of the fetal blood. Rh sensitization is the most common cause of Rh maternal immunization and

hemolysis of the fetal blood. A mother who is Rh negative and carrying an Rh-positive fetus is at risk of having a high-risk birth. This presence of anti-Rh_o (D) antibodies indicates the presence of an affected fetus. An antibody titer of above 1.8 is an indication that further evaluation must be done. RhoGam should be administered at approximately 28 weeks.

NP = An

CN = Ph/7

CL = An

SA = 3

12. 1. Fundal height in centimeters is approximately equal to weeks of gestation until the presenting part engages near term. Then the height decreases to approximately 38 cm. 35 cm is less than expected; 40 cm and 43 cm are more than expected.

NP = Ev

CN = He/3

CL = Ap

SA = 3

13. 2. A fetus that is longitudinal, cephalic lie, and in vertex presentation can deliver vaginally. Fetuses in a transverse position, longitudinal, cephalic lie, face presentation, and oblique lie must all deliver by cesarean section.

NP = Pl

CN = He/3

CL = Ap

SA = 3

14. 3. Presentation is the part of the fetus entering the pelvic inlet first. Terms used to identify this are shoulder, breech, and cephalic. Plus 3 means that the presenting part can be seen in the mother's perineum (station). The relationship of the long axis of the fetus to that of the mother is the fetal lie. The term includes longitudinal, transverse, and oblique. The relationship of the presenting part of the fetus to the ischial spines of the pelvis is position.

NP = Im

CN = He/3

CL = Ap

SA = 3

15. 4. By definition of the phases of the first stage of labor, a client who is 5 cm dilated is in active phase. Second stage begins with full dilatation of the cervix.

NP = Im

CN = He/3

CL = Ap

SA = 3

16. 1, 4, 6. A rigid, tender uterus, severe abdominal pain, and bright red bleeding describe abruptio placentae, a complication. A maternal urge to push, involuntary efforts, bulging of the perineum, and a visible fetal head at the introitus are all normal indications of imminent delivery.
NP = An
CN = He/3
CL = An
SA = 3

17. 3. As much as 80 to 90% of postpartum hemorrhage results from uterine atony. The nurse should assess the fundal height, fundal tone, lochia, and vital signs. The main clinical manifestation of a pelvic hematoma is pain unrelieved by analgesics. An elevated temperature would be present in an infection. Disseminated intravascular coagulation is related to systemic coagulopathies.
NP = As
CN = Ph/7
CL = An
SA = 3

18. 3. Relaxin causes connective tissue laxity. Estrogen, progesterone, and melantropin are increased in pregnancy, but do not affect connective tissue.
NP = Im
CN = He/3
CL = Ap
SA = 3

19. 3. Placing a hand on the client's shoulder and expressing sympathy communicate acceptance and understanding. Telling the mother that losing the fetus in utero is better than having seen the child invalidates the mother's grief. Regardless of gestation, the loss and grief are overwhelming. Telling the mother that it is God's will imposes the nurse's beliefs on the client. The client's belief system may be different from the nurse's. Avoidance of the client creates isolation and deprivation of support.
NP = An
CN = He/3
CL = An
SA = 3

Practice Test 2

1. The nurse understands that what pain control theory is responsible for decreasing the client's perception of pain after utilization of cutaneous stimulation, music, breathing, and hydrotherapy? _____

2. The nurse caring for a mother in labor who was sexually abused in childhood notes that the client is curled in a fetal position, sucking the thumb, and speaking in a childlike voice. The nurse documents this behavior as which of the following defense mechanisms?

   1. Displacement
   2. Regression
   3. Sublimation
   4. Introjection

3. Which of the following nursing actions is appropriate for a client who delivered vaginally three hours earlier and is complaining of excruciating vulvar pain?

   1. Inform the client that this is normal following an episiotomy
   2. Notify the physician
   3. Assess the fundus for tenderness
   4. Assess for uterine atony

4. The nurse is caring for a laboring mother in transition when the mother screams, "The baby's coming." The nurse inspects the perineum and sees that the fetal head is crowning. Which of the following interventions should the nurse perform?

   1. Ask the family to leave the room
   2. Promptly go to the nurses' station and call the physician

3. Administer intravenous pain medication per protocol to slow labor

4. Ask a staff member to notify the physician and stay with the client

5. During a delivery, the nurse notes that the fetal head pulls back instead of completing the external rotation process and progresses into the mother's pelvis. The nurse should notify the physician of which of the following?

1. Impending breech delivery

2. An android pelvis

3. The presence of shoulder dystocia

4. A transverse lie

6. When assisting in a delivery, which of the following interventions for a client presenting with a shoulder dystocia should the nurse implement?

1. Prepare for cesarean delivery

2. Apply fundal pressure

3. Apply suprapubic pressure

4. Administer muscle relaxants

7. Based on an understanding of the Rh factor in pregnancy, the nurse understands that a client who is a sensitized Rh-negative and has an Rh-positive infant is at high risk for developing what condition? _____

8. The registered nurse is delegating nursing tasks on a maternity unit. Which of the following nursing tasks should the nurse delegate to a licensed practical nurse?

1. Provide the care for a client suspected of having hydrops fetalis

2. Monitor the fetal tracings of a mother in labor

3. Apply the suprapubic pressure in a client presenting with shoulder dystonia

4. Provide comfort measures to a client who is 37 weeks of gestation

ANSWERS AND RATIONALES

1. **Gate control theory.** The gate control theory explains the relationship of pain and emotion. Stimulating cutaneous nerve fibers "closes the gate" to pain impulses. It has created a holistic nature to treating a client's pain.
NP = An
CN = He/3
CL = Ap
SA = 3

2. 2. Regression is retreating to a previous developmental state. Displacement is a transfer of feelings or reactions created by a specific topic or event to another that is less threatening. Sublimation channels

socially unacceptable behavior to socially acceptable behavior. Introjection incorporates without examining the thoughts of others as one's own.
NP = Im
CN = He/3
CL = Ap
SA = 3

3. 2. The client with a hematoma expresses excruciating pain and the physician should be notified. Severe pain is not normal following episiotomy. Fundal tenderness is associated with chorioamnionitis, uterine atony, or hemorrhage, not with hematoma of the vulva.
NP = Pl
CN = He/3
CL = Ap
SA = 3

4. 4. Sending the family out will deprive the woman of support and cause anxiety for the family. When delivery is imminent the nurse must stay at the bedside; leaving the room to call the physician is not appropriate. Pain medication should not be given when delivery is imminent because it can cause neonatal respiratory depression.
NP = Im
CN = He/3
CL = Ap
SA = 3

5. 3. The head would not emerge if the fetus were in a breech presentation or a transverse lie. The turtle sign describes the pulling back of the fetal head instead of completing the external rotation and progressing forward and is associated with shoulder dystocia. Android pelvis is associated with forceps and vacuum delivery.
NP = An
CN = He/3
CL = Ap
SA = 3

6. 3. A cesarean delivery is not indicated or practical for a client presenting with a shoulder dystocia. Fundal pressure is contraindicated in this situation; it worsens the impaction of the shoulder. Muscle relaxants are not used in this situation. Suprapubic pressure helps dislodge the shoulder and flexion and external rotation of the hips (McRobert's maneuver), increasing the pelvic diameters.
NP = Im
CN = He/3
CL = Ap
SA = 3

7. **Hydrops fetalis.** A sensitized Rh-negative client who has an Rh-positive fetus results in hemolysis of the fetal blood and hydrops fetalis may occur. In this condition, severe edema of the placenta and fetus occurs.The fetus may have cardiac and pleural effusions, cardiac enlargement, splenomegaly, and hepatomegaly.

NP = An
CN = He/3
CL = Ap
SA = 3

8. 4. It is appropriate to delegate providing comfort measures to a client who is 37 weeks of gestation to a licensed practical nurse. Caring for a client suspected of having hydrops fetalis, monitoring the fetal tracing of a mother in labor, and applying the suprapubic pressure to a client presenting with shoulder dystonia should all be delegated to a registered nurse.

NP = An
CN = Sa/1
CL = An
SA = 8

THE POSTPARTAL PERIOD - COMPREHENSIVE EXAM

1. Which of the following clinical manifestations would the nurse assess as indicative of pregnancy induced hypertension (PIH) in a client two days after vaginal delivery?

Select all that apply:

[ ] 1. Epigastric pain

[ ] 2. Ringing in the ears

[ ] 3. Chest pain

[ ] 4. Headache

[ ] 5. Visual changes

[ ] 6. Edema

2. A client who was diagnosed with GDM (gestational diabetes mellitus) asks the nurse what the chances are of having diabetes mellitus after the birth of the baby. Which of the following is the best response by the nurse?

1. "Gestational diabetes mellitus resolves in most women after pregnancy."

2. "Gestational diabetes mellitus is not a risk factor for the development of type 2 DM."

   3. "Once insulin is required, the pancreas will need a continued supply."
   4. "There is nothing you can do to prevent the onset of diabetes mellitus."

3. When the nurse is making a follow-up call to a client who delivered two weeks ago, the client expresses "feeling tearful, unhappy, and like a failure as a mother with no family support." Which of the following is the most appropriate intervention for this client? Instruct the client to

   1. see if she feels better in another week.
   2. ask a friend for help.
   3. come to the clinic for evaluation.
   4. get more sleep.

4. A postpartum client who delivered 24 hours ago informs the nurse of having night sweats but denies other complaints. The vital signs are: temperature 37.3°C, or 99.2°F; pulse, 68; respiratory rate, 18 beats per minute; and blood pressure, 120/68. Which of the following is the most appropriate intervention?

   1. Notify the physician
   2. Inform the client of the presence of an infection
   3. Continue to monitor the vital signs
   4. Inform the client this is a normal finding and continue to monitor

5. Methylergonovine maleate (Methergine) has been ordered for a postpartum client. The nurse should withhold this drug when which of the following is present?

   1. Uterine blood flow decreasing
   2. Tender breasts
   3. Pulse of 68
   4. Blood pressure of 145/96

6. Which of the following should the nurse include in the instructions about the use of narcotic pain medication following delivery?

   1. The pain medication will not be addicting
   2. Use the pain medication only when the pain is intense
   3. The pain medication may be constipating
   4. Driving is permitted while taking this medication

7. A postpartum client has many questions regarding care of herself and the infant. The nurse identifies which of the following nursing diagnoses to be the priority for this client?

   1. Pain
   2. Deficient knowledge

3. Activity intolerance

4. Ineffective infant feeding pattern

8. Which of the following interventions should the nurse include in the plan of care for a client experiencing hemorrhoidal pain postpartum?

1. Decrease fiber in the diet

2. Decrease activity

3. Fleets enema

4. Tucks pads and ice packs to the area

9. A client asks the nurse if there are calories in colostrum. The appropriate response by the nurse is that colostrum

1. "has more calories per ounce than breast milk."

2. "has fewer calories per ounce than breast milk."

3. "is very comparable in calories with breast milk."

4. "has no calories."

10. The nurse should instruct a client in the postpartum period to perform which of the following exercises to strengthen the pelvic floor muscles?

1. Sit-ups

2. Push-ups

3. Kegel exercises

4. Lunges

11. Six hours after delivery, the nurse should administer how much insulin to a client who has gestational diabetes mellitus?

1. An increased amount from the predelivery amount

2. No insulin is needed

3. The same amount of insulin as used during pregnancy

4. Change to oral diabetic medications

12. The nurse informs a client in the postpartum period that a noninvasive test measuring electric resistance and blood flow in the veins of the legs to diagnose deep vein thrombosis is

1. an impedance plethysmography.

2. a duplex ultrasonography.

3. a spiral CT scan.

4. a V/Q scan.

13. The nurse should monitor a postpartum client for which of the following complications that causes one third of all the maternal deaths in the postpartum period?

1. Hematoma
2. Hemorrhage
3. Infection
4. Deep vein thrombus

14. The nurse is caring for a client admitted with thrombophlebitis. The nurse should assess a client for which of the following clinical manifestations of thrombophlebitis?
Select all that apply:

[ ] 1. Pain

[ ] 2. Edema of the area

[ ] 3. Positive Homan's sign

[ ] 4. Increased bowel sounds

[ ] 5. Cool and pale extremity

[ ] 6. Bradycardia

15. The nurse is assessing the following four postpartum clients for being at risk of developing a hematoma. Which of the following postpartum clients does the nurse evaluate as being at greatest risk?

1. A client who delivered a 6 lb infant in 6 hours
2. A client who delivered an 8 lb infant with a forceps delivery
3. A client who had 5 lb twins
4. A client who delivered a 7 lb infant after 14 hours of labor

16. On the second postpartum day, a client states that she has voided four times in the last two hours. The nurse should initially

1. call the physician.
2. assess the client's fluid intake.
3. measure the client's next voided urine.
4. instruct the client to decrease fluid intake.

17. The nurse is assessing a client after delivery and finds the uterine fundus boggy and one centimeter above the umbilicus. Which of the following is the priority nursing intervention?

1. Assess the vital signs
2. Massage the uterus
3. Assess the perineal area
4. Notify the physician

18. A client diagnosed with mastitis is concerned that her infant will be infected if she continues to breast-feed. Which of the following is the appropriate response by the nurse?

1. "You are correct and need to stop breastfeeding."
2. "The bacteria are localized in the breast tissue and do not enter the breast milk."
3. "The infant received immunity through the breast milk and is not susceptible."
4. "The infant will need to be started on an antibiotic also."

19. The nurse assesses the vaginal flow on the perineal pad of a postpartum client to be covering a three-inch area in the past hour. In determining what action to take next, which of the following should the nurse consider? This amount of vaginal flow is considered a

1. scant flow.
2. light flow.
3. moderate flow.
4. heavy flow.

20. The nurse assesses a client to have a positive Homan's sign. What is the clinical manifestation the nurse evaluates this client to have? _____

21. The nurse should perform which of the following nursing actions when a client with pre-eclampsia has a seizure in the postpartum period? Select all that apply:

[ ] 1. Stay with the client

[ ] 2. Insert a tongue blade in the client's mouth

[ ] 3. Administer oxygen

[ ] 4. Position to prevent aspiration

[ ] 5. Give hydantoin (Dilantin) IV push stat

[ ] 6. Restrain the client

22. The client phones the clinic and tells the nurse that after discharge from the hospital following a vaginal delivery, the swelling is worse in her legs than before discharge. The appropriate response by the nurse is

1. "The edema should have resolved by the day of discharge."
2. "Kidney function is adequate and lower extremity edema is not a concern."
3. "Lower extremity edema may become worse after discharge."
4. "Edema persisting after discharge should be treated with a diuretic."

23. A client two days after a cesarean section is experiencing increased abdominal pain, prolonged and severe cramping, and a malodorous discharge. The nurse should notify the physician that the client is experiencing a postpartum infection of _____ .

24. A postpartum client who is attempting breastfeeding is worried that her breasts are small. The nurse's best response is

1. "The size of your breasts will not affect your ability to feed your baby."

2. "I am sure you will do fine."

3. "Women find that the baby cannot latch on when their breasts are small."

4. "You should plan to supplement."

25. Which of the following should the nurse include when teaching postpartum nurses about thyrotoxic storm in a postpartum client?

1. Thyrotoxic storm is caused by a deficit in the thyroid hormone

2. Thyrotoxic storm is often confused with postpartum depression

3. Thyrotoxic storm is a life-threatening emergency

4. The client's thyroid is not damaged following a thyrotoxic storm

26. The registered nurse is planning the clinical assignments on a postpartum maternity unit. Which of the following nursing skills should the nurse delegate to a licensed practical nurse?

1. Care for a client who is experiencing a thyrotoxic storm

2. Instruct a client on the clinical manifestations of eclampsia

3. Administer a pain medication to a client experiencing pain following delivery

4. Monitor a client for postpartal hemorrhage

ANSWERS AND RATIONALES

1. 1, 4, 5, 6. Pregnancy induced hypertension can extend into the postpartum period. Cardinal clinical manifestations include headache, visual changes, proteinuria, hypertension, epigastric pain, and edema.
NP = As
CN = He/3
CL = Ap
SA = 3

2. 1. Gestational diabetes mellitus will resolve in most women, but the client will be at risk for developing type 2 diabetes mellitus later in life. The client can delay or prevent the onset of type 2 diabetes mellitus with proper diet and exercise.
NP = An
CN = He/3
CL = An
SA = 3

3. 3. It is very important to diagnose postpartum depression early so that the maternal-child relationship is allowed to proceed and develop in a positive way. Drugs and frequent follow-up visits are also useful in treating this disorder. It is important to get the client back in the health care system for evaluation as soon as possible.
NP = Pl
CN = He/3
CL = Ap
SA = 3

4. 4. Diaphoresis is common after delivery, especially at night. It is the body's way to rid itself of excessive fluids no longer needed after delivery.
NP = Pl
CN = He/3
CL = Ap
SA = 3

5. 4. Methylergonovine maleate (Methergine) is an oxytocin drug used in the treatment of postpartum hemorrhage. It should not be given to a hypertensive client whose blood pressure is elevated, because this medication also elevates blood pressure.
NP = Im
CN = Ph/6
CL = Ap
SA = 5

6. 3. An adverse reaction to pain medication is constipation; a postpartum client often fears her first bowel movement after delivery, so it is important to let her know about this. Narcotics can be addictive if used long term. Waiting until the pain is intense is counter-effective. It should be used with the onset of pain to keep it at an acceptable level. Driving is not permitted while taking pain medication.
NP = Pl
CN = He/3
CL = Ap
SA = 3

7. 2. Asking many questions in regard to infant care necessitates the need for opening a deficient knowledge diagnosis.
NP = An
CN = He/3
CL = Ap
SA = 3

8. 4. Ice would help reduce the swelling and numb the area around hemorrhoids. Tucks pads help soothe and shrink hemorrhoidal tissue. It

is important to increase fiber in the diet to prevent constipation. Decreased activity leads to constipation. A Fleets enema would be an extreme measure and would cause more irritation to the area.
NP = Im
CN = He/3
CL = Ap
SA = 3

9. 3. Colostrum is a rich, concentrated form of early breast milk that is high in calories and antibodies and comparable to the calories in breast milk.
NP = An
CN = He/3
CL = An
SA = 3

10. 3. Kegel exercises are extremely important after delivery. This exercise helps the postpartum client regain muscle tone that was lost due to stretching and loss of tone during the delivery process. Sit-ups, push-ups, and lunges are all exercises, but they don't strengthen the pelvic floor muscles.
NP = Pl
CN = He/3
CL = Ap
SA = 3

11. 2. The insulin requirements diminish precipitously and it is often unnecessary to give insulin after delivery to the client who had gestational diabetes mellitus. Gestational diabetes mellitus usually resolves after delivery, so no drug therapy is needed.
NP = Im
CN = Ph/6
CL = Ap
SA = 5

12. 1. Impedance plethysmography is a safe, noninvasive, and reasonable specific test for proximal deep vein thrombosis, measuring impedance or electrical resistance in blood flow caused by clots. Duplex ultrasonography is a test that measures disruption of blood flow. Spiral CT scan and V/Q scan are both tests used to diagnose pulmonary emboli.
NP = Im
CN = Ph/7
CL = Co
SA = 3

13. 2. The incidence of hemorrhage is very high. Predisposing factors are very important to assess for in the postpartum client. Early intervention

provides optimum outcomes. Hematoma, infection, and deep vein thrombosis are complications that rarely cause mortality.
NP = As
CN = Ph/7
CL = An
SA = 3

14. 1, 2, 3. Thrombophlebitis occurs in less than 1% of the postpartum population. Physical findings are important to identify in order to prevent the increased risk of pulmonary embolism, which could lead to death in the postpartum client. Clinical manifestations include pain, tachycardia, decreased bowel sounds, redness and warm tenderness in the calves, and a positive Homan's sign.
NP = As
CN = He/3
CL = Ap
SA = 3

15. 2. Trauma from forceps manipulation poses the greatest risk in the formation of a hematoma. A client who delivered a 6 lb infant in 6 hours, a client who had twins, and a client who delivered a 7 lb infant after 14 hours of labor would all be at very low risk for the formation of a hematoma.
NP = Ev
CN = Ph/7
CL = An
SA = 3

16. 3. Urinary retention may occur due to edema and trauma from the delivery process. Output must be assessed before other interventions are applicable. More data must be obtained before reporting.
NP = Im
CN = He/3
CL = Ap
SA = 3

17. 2. It is very important that the uterine fundus remains firm after delivery so that bleeding is controlled. Although assessing the vital signs and perineal area may be appropriate, they are not the priority. Notifying the physician would be appropriate only after massaging the uterus.
NP = Pl
CN = Sa/1
CL = Ap
SA = 3

18. 2. Organisms that cause mastitis do not enter the breast milk. Mastitis is not contraindicated with breastfeeding and breastfeeding may be continued. Even though the baby does receive antibodies through the

breast milk, the milk is not infected with mastitis. Bacteria do not enter the breast milk.

NP = An
CN = He/3
CL = An
SA = 3

19. 2. Light flow is defined as less than a four-inch stain in one hour. A scant flow is less than a one-inch stain in one hour. A stain less than six inches in one hour is considered a moderate flow. Heavy flow is a saturated pad in one hour.

NP = An
CN = He/3
CL = Ap
SA = 3

20. Pain with dorsiflexion of the foot. A positive Homan's sign is pain up the back of the leg with dorsiflexion of the foot.

NP = Ev
CN = He/3
CL = Co
SA = 3

21. 1, 3, 4. Staying with the client, administering oxygen, and positioning the client to prevent aspiration are appropriate measures that attempt to ensure the client's safety and maintain airway integrity during a seizure in a client with pre-eclampsia. Inserting a tongue blade in the client's mouth is no longer recommended because it may cause harm as long as the client has a patent airway. If the client loses the airway during the seizure, a tongue blade is not adequate because the client is in respiratory arrest. Magnesium sulfate is the drug of choice to quiet the central nervous system for pre-eclamptic clients who have seizures rather than hydantoin (Dilantin).

NP = Pl
CN = He/3
CL = Ap
SA = 3

22. 3. Edema in the extremities may become worse once the postpartum client is home from the hospital since the client is up on her feet more. Some edema may be present normally after discharge. Edema (unilateral) may be a sign of deep vein thrombosis and is not always benign, but it would not require diuretic medication.

NP = An
CN = He/3
CL = An
SA = 3

23. the uterus. A uterine infection occurs one to three days after a cesarean section with clinical manifestations of severe cramping, increased abdominal pain, and a malodorous discharge being classic.
NP = An
CN = He/3
CL = An
SA = 3

24. 1. Breast size does not affect the ability to produce milk.
NP = An
CN = He/3
CL = An
SA = 3

25. 3. Thyrotoxic storm is a state of increased thyroid activity from excessive thyroid hormones and is life threatening. Metabolic functions are sped up. Of women who develop thyroiditis, 10 to 30% develop permanent hypothyroidism.
NP = Pl
CN = He/3
CL = An
SA = 3

26. 3. A licensed practical nurse may administer a pain medication to a client experiencing pain following delivery. A client who is experiencing a thyrotoxic storm should be cared for by a registered nurse because it is life threatening. Instructing a client about the clinical manifestations of eclampsia and monitoring a client for postpartal hemorrhage should be performed by a registered nurse.
NP = Pl
CN = Sa/1
CL = An
SA = 3

NEWBORN CARE - COMPREHENSIVE EXAM

1. When caring for a newborn whose mother had oliguria for several weeks during pregnancy, the nurse should assess the newborn for what disorder? _____

2. The nurse assesses the development of a slight yellow tinge to the skin of a 2-day-old newborn. Which of the following is the priority intervention?

1. Instruct the mother to discontinue breastfeeding
2. Obtain a serum bilirubin level
3. Report this as an obstructive intestinal process
4. Report this as a sign of physiologic jaundice

3. The nurse evaluates a 12-hour-old newborn who is blood type AB-negative and who has a mother with type O blood. The nurse assesses the newborn to have a marked yellow tinge to the skin. The nurse should report this as

   1. breastfeeding jaundice.
   2. Rh-isoimmunization.
   3. pathological jaundice.
   4. physiologic jaundice.

4. The nurse evaluates a newborn immediately after birth to have a heart rate of 90, blue skin color, no response to a catheter in the naris, no respiratory effort, and no muscle tone. The nurse should document the Apgar as

   1. 3.
   2. 5.
   3. 2.
   4. 1.

5. At five minutes of age, a newborn has a heart rate of 130, is acrocyanotic, grimaces in response to a catheter in the naris, has a respiratory rate of 30 with good air exchange, and is able to flex all extremities. Which of the following is the correct five-minute Apgar documentation?

   1. 10
   2. 7
   3. 6
   4. 9

6. Based on an understanding of the various types of deliveries, for which of the following deliveries is it a priority to have resuscitation personnel available?

   1. Cesarean delivery
   2. Premature birth delivery
   3. All deliveries
   4. Multiple gestation delivery

7. During a newborn assessment, the parents ask the nurse what is the downy hair on several areas of the body of the newborn. The nurse informs the parents that this is _____ .

8. The nurse documents a cheesy material in the skin folds of the neck and groin of a newborn during physical examination as _____ .

9. A mother asks the nurse to see the "bug bites" on her newborn, and asks how insects could have bitten her infant while in the hospital nursery. Which of the following is the appropriate response by the nurse?

   1. "These are the result of a candidiasis infection and are treated with a topical antifungal."

   2. "This is a benign self-limiting condition called erythema toxicum neonatorum."

   3. "I will notify the physician of the bug bites on your newborn."

   4. "Bullous impetigo consists of bullous vesicular lesions treated with an oral antibiotic."

10. The parents of a newborn ask the nurse to look at the blood on their uncircumcised son's diaper. The nurse informs the parents that these salmon or peach stains on the diaper are normal in the first few days of life and consist of

    1. blood.

    2. iron.

    3. casts.

    4. uric acid crystals.

11. The nurse is assisting a new mother to breast-feed her newborn. The mother asks the nurse how to know if the baby is getting anything from the breast. The nurse should inform the mother that the best indication that the newborn is getting breast milk is which of the following?

    1. Audible swallowing

    2. Burping

    3. Sucking in short bursts with short rest periods between bursts

    4. Sleeping for five hours after a feeding

ANSWERS AND RATIONALES

1. **Pulmonary hypoplasia.** Pulmonary hypoplasia is a disorder that occurs in infants whose mother had oliguria for several weeks during pregnancy.
   NP = As
   CN = He/3
   CL = Ap
   SA = 3

2. **4.** Physiologic jaundice appears on the second to third day, peaks on the third or fourth day, and gradually decreases between the fifth and seventh days. Jaundice that appears on the fifth to seventh day may be breast milk

jaundice. Jaundice within the first 24 hours of life is pathological jaundice and the result of hemolytic disease.

NP = Im
CN = He/3
CL = Ap
SA = 3

3. 3. Pathological jaundice appears before 24 hours and increases sharply. This newborn is at risk for ABO incompatibility, but not for Rh-isoimmunization. Physiologic jaundice develops more slowly. Breastfeeding jaundice appears on the fifth to seventh day of life.

NP = An
CN = Ph/7
CL = An
SA = 3

4. 4. The infant has an Apgar score of 1 when there is a pulse below 100 beats per minute with no points given for the other areas. The Apgar test is a numerical expression of the well-being of the newborn. The score is assigned to the newborn at 1, 5, and 15 minutes. The other Apgar areas are respiratory effort, heart rate, muscle tone, reflex irritability, and color. This newborn requires resuscitation.

NP = Im
CN = He/3
CL = An
SA = 3

5. 4. The Apgar test is a numerical expression of the well-being of the newborn. The score is assigned to the newborn at 1, 5, and 15 minutes. The other Apgar areas are respiratory effort, heart rate, muscle tone, reflex irritability, and color. Each of the Apgar assessment criteria is equal to 2 points, with the exception of a 1-point deduction for the acrocyanosis, to give an Apgar score of 9. This is a normal Apgar score. Apgar scores between 7 and 10 indicate the newborn is able to adjust to extrauterine life without difficulty.

NP = Im
CN = He/3
CL = Ap
SA = 3

6. 3. Although cesarean, multiple gestation, and premature birth deliveries have an increased risk for resuscitation, resuscitation personnel should be available at all deliveries to anticipate the unknown.

NP = An
CN = Ph/7
CL = An
SA = 3

7. lanugo. Lanugo is the downy hair present on the body of the fetus between the 20th week of gestation and birth.
NP = Im
CN = He/3
CL = Ap
SA = 3

8. vernix caseosa. Vernix caseosa consists of desquamated epithelial cells and sebum, protects the skin, and aids thermal stability. It appears as a cheesy material in the skin folds usually found in the neck and groin.
NP = Im
CN = He/3
CL = Ap
SA = 3

9. 2. Erythema toxicum neonatorum, also called "fleabite dermatitis" or "newborn rash," is a transient maculopapular condition. It generally appears on the second or third day of life. They are small, 1 to 3 mm, pale yellow, and firm lesions that resemble flea bites. The etiology is unknown and no treatment is required. Parents need to be assured that this is a benign condition.
NP = An
CN = He/3
CL = An
SA = 3

10. 4. Uric acid crystals may appear in the concentrated urine of a newborn. They may appear as salmon or peach stains on the diaper of an uncircumcised male. Females or circumcised males could have blood in the diaper. Iron or casts would not appear in the diaper.
NP = An
CN = He/3
CL = Ap
SA = 3

11. 1. Audible swallowing is the best indication that an infant is getting something from the breast. Short bursts of sucking, followed by a rest period, is a normal newborn feeding pattern, but does not indicate adequate intake. Breast-fed newborns do not normally sleep for five hours after a feeding. Burping is not related to milk intake.
NP = Im
CN = He/3
CL = Ap
SA = 3

Practice Test 3

NEWBORN CARE - COMPREHENSIVE EXAM

1. A mother who is HIV positive and in labor is preparing to deliver. Which of the following drugs should the nurse prepare for immediate administration in the delivery room?
   1. Vitamin K
   2. Erythromycin eye ointment
   3. Zidovudine (Retrovir)
   4. Ampicillin

2. The nurse is preparing to initiate bottle-feeding in a 2-hour-old, 36-week-gestation newborn. Which of the following findings would be an indication to delay the feeding and notify the physician?
   1. Temperature of 36.8°C, or 98.2°F axillary
   2. Pulse of 130
   3. Acrocyanosis
   4. Respiratory rate of 78

3. Two hours after birth, the nurse is caring for an irritable and jittery infant of a mother who has diabetes mellitus. Which of the following should the nurse assess?
   1. Temperature
   2. Blood pressure
   3. Bilirubin
   4. Blood sugar

4. Which of the following should the nurse include in the plan of care for a narcotic-exposed newborn who is crying and is difficult to console?

1. Play soothing music in the newborn's environment
2. Place the newborn in a quiet and dimly lighted area
3. Sing a lullaby to the newborn
4. Position the newborn in a crib with colorful mobiles

5. What clinical assessment scale is a priority for the nurse to use to perform a gestational age assessment? _____

6. The nurse is caring for a newborn 15 minutes after birth. The newborn's color is pale, mottled, has decreased muscle tone, and a prolonged capillary refill. Which of the following is a priority for the nurse to assess in this infant?
   1. Breath sounds
   2. Blood pressure
   3. Bowel sounds
   4. Chest circumference

7. The nurse is caring for a newborn with an infection. After reviewing the delivery history, the nurse evaluates which of the following as the most likely cause of the infection?
   1. Rupture of membranes for 28 hours
   2. Precipitous delivery
   3. Cesarean birth
   4. Use of forceps

8. When preparing to care for a newborn with poor muscle tone, the nurse should plan on an increased heat loss due to the loss of which heat conservation mechanism?
   1. Flexed position
   2. Peripheral vasodilatation
   3. Limited subcutaneous fat
   4. Large body surface–to-weight ratio

9. The parents of an African-American newborn express concern to the nurse about the bluish hyperpigmented spots on the newborn's sacral area. The nurse informs the parents that these spots are a normal finding called
   1. Koplik's spots.
   2. Epstein's pearls.
   3. mongolian spots.
   4. erythema toxicum neonatorum.

10. The nurse is caring for a newborn with white inclusion cysts in the mouth. The nurse documents these as _____ .

11. A mother asks the nurse in to look at her newborn's rash. When the nurse goes to look at the rash, it has disappeared. The nurse should inform the mother that the rash that disappeared is which of the following?

   1. Koplik's spots

   2. Epstein's pearls

   3. Mongolian spots

   4. Erythema toxicum neonatorum

12. The nurse is observing another nurse administer intramuscular injections to a newborn. Which of the following sites indicates the nurse is administering the intramuscular injections in the correct site?

   1. Vastus lateralis

   2. Deltoid

   3. Ventrogluteal

   4. Gluteal

13. The nurse assesses the singing, moaning, and whining sounds with each expiration that a newborn is experiencing as the result of an increased respiratory effort and reports it as

   1. retractions.

   2. nasal flaring.

   3. grunting.

   4. reflux.

14. When reviewing the delivery history of a newborn, the nurse notes that the mother tested positive for cocaine at several prenatal visits. The nurse should monitor this newborn for which of the following?

   1. Abstinence syndrome

   2. Abnormal facies

   3. Respiratory depression

   4. Irritability and inability to calm

15. Which of the following goals should the nurse include in the plan of care for a newborn during the first six hours of life?

   1. Void at least once

   2. Pass meconium

   3. Maintain heart rate between 110 and 160 beats per minute

   4. Maintain respiratory rate between 12 and 20 breaths per minute

16. Immediately following delivery, the nurse dries the newborn thoroughly to prevent heat loss by _____ .

17. After assessing a score of zero on a newborn using the Silverman-Anderson index, the nurse should

    1. notify the physician.
    2. call the respiratory therapist.
    3. administer oxygen.
    4. continue to monitor the newborn.

18. The nurse evaluates a bluish color to the hands and feet of a 3-hour-old newborn. The nurse documents this as _____ .

19. The registered nurse is preparing to delegate nursing tasks on a newborn care unit. Which of the following tasks should the nurse delegate to a licensed practical nurse?

    1. Administer an intramuscular injection to a newborn
    2. Assess a newborn for phenylketonuria
    3. Perform a gestational age assessment
    4. Monitor the laboratory data in a premature infant

ANSWERS AND RATIONALES

1. 3. Zidovudine (Retrovir) is an antiviral used to prevent HIV transmission from pregnant women to their fetuses. The newborn should receive Retrovir in the delivery room to minimize the likelihood of HIV or AIDS. Vitamin K is used as a prophylaxis and therapy of hemorrhagic disease. Erythromycin is used as a prophylaxis for sexually transmitted diseases. While vitamin K and eye prophylaxis are generally given within one hour of delivery, Retrovir should be given in the first minutes of life. Ampicillin is not given immediately after delivery.
   NP = Im
   CN = Ph/6
   CL = Ap
   SA = 5

2. 4. The respiratory rate of a newborn should be below 60 breaths per minute. A respiratory rate above 60 breaths per minute would compromise the newborn's ability to suck-swallow-breathe. A respiratory rate of 78 breaths per minute is tachypnea. Normal axillary temperature is between $36.5°C$ and $37.6°C$, or $97.7°F$ and $99.7°F$. The normal pulse rate is between 130 and 160 beats per minute. Acrocyanosis is normal and usually present in the feet and hands.

NP = An
CN = He/3
CL = Ap
SA = 3

3. 4. Infants experience a hyperinsulin state in utero and are at risk for hypoglycemia. Hypoglycemia may cause jitters and eventually seizures. Variations in vital signs do not cause jitters. It is unlikely that hemolysis is sufficient to affect bilirubin by two hours of age.
NP = As
CN = He/3
CL = Ap
SA = 3

4. 2. Minimizing sensory stimulation is essential for a narcotic-exposed newborn, due to hyperirritability and an inability to tune out stimuli. Placing the newborn in a dimly lighted and quiet environment would decrease sensory stimuli.
NP = Pl
CN = He/3
CL = Ap
SA = 3

5. Dubowitz scale and Ballard scale. The Dubowitz scale assesses six external physical and six neuromuscular signs. The cumulative score correlates with a maturity rating for a gestational age between 35 to 42 weeks. The Ballard scale measures the same physical and neuromuscular signs, but also includes 1 to 2 signs in premature infants. It may be used on newborns as young as 20 weeks of gestation.
NP = Im
CN = He/3
CL = Ap
SA = 3

6. 1. Poor cardiac output in the newborn is almost always related to respiratory insufficiency or distress. Hypotension is a late sign of cardiopulmonary compromise. The nurse should assess breath sounds first, and proceed based on that assessment.
NP = As
CN = He/3
CL = Ap
SA = 3

7. 1. Rupture of membranes for more than 24 hours increases the risk of infection significantly. The use of forceps or precipitous delivery should

alert the nurse to assess for birth trauma. A cesarean birth triggers the need to assess for transient tachypnea of the newborn.

NP = Ev
CN = He/3
CL = Ap
SA = 3

8. 1. A flexed position decreases heat loss. A loss of this mechanism would increase heat loss. Peripheral vasodilation, limited subcutaneous fat, and large body surface-to-weight ratio also increase the heat loss, but are not related to poor muscle tone.

NP = Pl
CN = He/3
CL = An
SA = 3

9. 3. Mongolian spots are a dark blue, gray, or purple color seen on the buttocks. Koplik's spots are irregular and small red spots with small bluish white centers that appear on the buccal mucosa. They are seen in measles (rubeola) before the appearance of a rash. Epstein's pearls are small white epithelial cysts found on the hard palate and considered a normal finding. Erythema toxicum neonatorum produces small pale yellow lesions that resemble flea bites and is a normal transient maculopapular condition.

NP = Im
CN = He/3
CL = Ap
SA = 3

10. Epstein's pearls. Epstein's pearls are small white epithelial cysts found on the hard palate and are considered a normal finding.

NP = Im
CN = He/3
CL = Co
SA = 3

11. 4. Blanched plaques on erythematous bases that appear and disappear rapidly are characteristic of erythema toxicum neonatorum. Mongolian spots are a dark blue, gray, or purple color seen on the buttocks. Koplik's spots are irregular and small red spots with small bluish white centers that appear on the buccal mucosa. They are seen in measles (rubeola) before the appearance of a rash. Epstein's pearls are small white epithelial cysts found on the hard palate and are considered a normal finding. Koplik's spots, Epstein's pearls, and mongolian spots do not disappear rapidly.

NP = Im
CN = He/3

CL = Ap
SA = 3

12. 1. Newborn intramuscular injections are always given in the vastus lateralis. The deltoid, ventrogluteal, and gluteal sites are underdeveloped in the newborn and intramuscular injections in these sites pose a risk of injury to nerves and blood vessels.
NP = Ev
CN = Ph/7
CL = Ap
SA = 3

13. 3. Singing, moaning, and whining sounds with each expiration are characteristically found in grunting. While retractions and nasal flaring also reflect respiratory problems, these are noted on inspection. Reflux is not audible.
NP = An
CN = He/3
CL = An
SA = 3

14. 4. Abstinence syndrome and respiratory depression are associated with narcotic exposure. Abnormal facies are associated with alcohol exposure. Newborns exposed to cocaine are difficult to console and cannot tolerate usual interventions, such as rocking.
NP = As
CN = He/3
CL = Ap
SA = 3

15. 3. A heart rate of 110 to 160 is normal. The newborn is expected to void by 24 hours of age and pass meconium by 48 hours of age. The respiratory rate of 12 to 20 is not normal for a newborn. The respiratory rate should be approximately 60 breaths per minute. A respiratory rate between 12 and 20 is severe bradycardia. It is the normal respiratory rate for adults.
NP = Ev
CN = He/3
CL = An
SA = 3

16. evaporation. Drying the newborn prevents heat loss by evaporation.
NP = Im
CN = He/3
CL = Ap
SA = 3

17. 4. The score of zero on the Silverman-Anderson index indicates no respiratory depression. No action is necessary at this time. The nurse should continue to monitor the infant.
NP = Im
CN = He/3
CL = An
SA = 3

18. acrocyanosis. Acrocyanosis is a normal finding and not an indication of abnormal respiration or respiratory distress. It is normal in newborns and present on the hands and feet.
NP = Im
CN = He/3
CL = Co
SA = 3

19. 1. A licensed practical nurse may administer an intramuscular injection to a newborn. Assessing a newborn for phenylketonuria, performing a gestational assessment, and monitoring laboratory data are all tasks that require the skills of a registered nurse.
NP = Pl
CN = Sa/1
CL = An
SA = 8

REPRODUCTIVE DISORDERS - COMPREHENSIVE EXAM

1. The client who had a laparoscopy the day before asks the nurse, "Why do I have pain in my shoulders?" Which of the following is the best response by the nurse?

   1. "It's caused by the position you were placed in during the procedure."

   2. "It's a result of tensed muscles, because you were so anxious before the procedure."

   3. "It's referred pain from moving your pelvic organs during the procedure."

   4. "It's due to a gas injected during the procedure, which moves to your shoulders."

2. The nurse is taking a health history of a client with gonorrhea. Which of the following questions should the nurse ask that would affect the results of a cervical culture?

   1. "When was your last menstrual period?"

   2. "Have you douched within the last two hours?"

3. "Have you had sexual intercourse within the last 24 hours?"

4. "Do you think you might be pregnant?"

3. The nurse would note which of the following in the assessment of a client who is in the beginning stages of menopause (perimenopausal)?

   1. Painful intercourse

   2. Weight loss

   3. Amenorrhea

   4. Moist skin

4. The nurse should include which of the following in the instructions to the menopausal woman regarding ways to minimize the development of osteoporosis?

   1. Take vitamin B_6 and vitamin E supplements daily in the a.m.

   2. Develop hobbies that will minimize stress on your joints

   3. Exercise on a regular basis by walking at a fast pace

   4. Follow your physician's orders for taking progesterone each month

5. A thin, young female athlete asks the nurse, "Why don't I have regular periods like other girls my age?" The best reply of the nurse would be

   1. "Reduced body fat suppresses menstruation."

   2. "Increased muscle tone affects your hormone levels."

   3. "Exercise postpones the maturation of your female organs."

   4. "Changing your exercise program should restore your hormone balance."

6. Which of the following instructions should the nurse give a client experiencing dysmenorrhea?

   1. Take frequent hot showers

   2. Increase salt and fluid intake

   3. Take the prescribed muscle relaxants

   4. Exercise more frequently

7. The nurse instructs a client with premenstrual syndrome (PMS) to avoid which of the following foods when experiencing clinical manifestations of bloating and edema?
   Select all that apply:

   [ ] 1. Raw parsley

   [ ] 2. Cantaloupe

   [ ] 3. Applesauce

   [ ] 4. Asparagus

[ ] **5.** Broccoli

[ ] **6.** Celery

8. The nurse assesses a client with menorrhagia to have which of the following?

    1. Vaginal bleeding between regular menstrual periods

    2. Pain with sexual intercourse

    3. Prolonged or excessive vaginal bleeding with menses

    4. Pain with the beginning of menstrual flow

9. Which of the following goals would be most important to include in the teaching plan for the client with a rectovaginal fistula? The client will

    1. have optimal physical mobility.

    2. be free of infection.

    3. verbalize a positive body image.

    4. report decreased abdominal pain.

10. The client with a rectovaginal fistula asks the nurse what she can do to prevent the fistula from getting larger. The most appropriate response by the nurse is which of the following?

    1. "Increase your fluid intake to 8 to 10 glasses of water a day."

    2. "Eat foods that are high in fiber."

    3. "Take the prescribed paregoric after each bowel movement."

    4. "Change the vaginal tampon every three to four hours."

11. The nurse instructs a client to use what solution for a deodorizing douche?_____

12. The nurse is caring for a client with a cystocele. Which of the following assessment findings would the nurse evaluate as an anticipated finding?

    1. Stress incontinence

    2. Bloody urine

    3. Constipation

    4. Hemorrhoids

13. The nurse develops a plan of care for a postoperative client who had a cystocele repair (anterior colporrhaphy). The plan should include measures to monitor

    1. restricted movement for 24 hours.

    2. intake and output every 8 hours.

    3. vaginal bleeding every 3 to 4 hours.

    4. vital signs every 4 hours.

14. Which of the following is the most appropriate response when a client with a cystocele asks the nurse, "Why do I need to do Kegel exercises?"
    1. "It tightens your pelvic organs."
    2. "It will help to improve your stress incontinence."
    3. "It will alleviate the pelvic pain you're having."
    4. "It will strengthen your abdominal muscles."

15. The nurse is caring for a client who had an anterior and posterior colporrhaphy. Which of the following assessment findings would the nurse evaluate as a complication of this type of surgery?
    1. Complaints of pelvic cramping
    2. No bowel movement for two days
    3. Vaginal bleeding and clots
    4. Drainage from the abdominal incision

16. A client with a pessary asks the nurse why the pessary is used. The nurse informs the client that a pessary is used in the treatment of what condition?_____

17. Which of the following nursing diagnoses would be most appropriate for the client who douches frequently?
    1. Risk for infection
    2. Risk for impaired skin integrity
    3. Risk for urge incontinence
    4. Sexual dysfunction

18. The nurse assesses a client with candidiasis to have which of the following vaginal discharges?
    1. Thick yellow with purulent consistency
    2. Thick with cottage cheese consistency
    3. Gray with fishlike odor
    4. Thin yellow-brown with offensive odor

19. The nurse develops a plan of care for the client admitted with acute pelvic inflammatory disease. Which of the following interventions would be appropriate to incorporate into this client's plan of care?
    Select all that apply:
    [ ] 1. Apply a heat lamp to the perineum
    [ ] 2. Administer prescribed antibiotics
    [ ] 3. Instruct the client in the procedure for vinegar douche
    [ ] 4. Monitor amount, color, and consistency of vaginal bleeding

[   ] **5.** Instruct the client on safe sex practices

[   ] **6.** Maintain client on bed rest in semi-Fowler's position

20. The nurse is caring for a client with toxic shock syndrome. Which of the following would indicate to the nurse that the client's condition is deteriorating?

   1. Temperature of 38.9°C, or 102°F

   2. Unresponsive to verbal stimuli

   3. Complaints of severe muscle pain

   4. Blood pressure of 105/70

21. During an admission history, the nurse evaluates which of the following to be present in a client with uterine fibroids?
Select all that apply:

[   ] **1.** Low abdominal pressure

[   ] **2.** Menorrhagia

[   ] **3.** Spotting between periods

[   ] **4.** Dyspareunia

[   ] **5.** Backache

[   ] **6.** Constipation

22. The nurse should report which of the following assessments when caring for a postoperative client who had an abdominal hysterectomy?

   1. Faint bowel sounds

   2. Serosanguineous drainage in suction apparatus at the surgical site

   3. Several episodes of vomiting

   4. Vaginal bleeding

23. Which of the following should the nurse include in the instructions given to a client with endometriosis?

   1. Once the uterine bleeding is controlled, the clinical manifestations will disappear

   2. Pregnancy will provide relief from the pain you are experiencing

   3. As you get older, the episodes of pain will decrease in severity

   4. Exercise, good nutrition, and adequate rest will alleviate your clinical manifestations

24. The nurse evaluates a client with an ectopic pregnancy to have which of the following?

   1. BP of 80/50

   2. Thick mucus vaginal discharge

3. Difficulty in voiding

4. Complaints of dragging pain in pelvis and back

25. Which of the following should the nurse include in the discharge instructions given to a client after treatment for an ectopic pregnancy?

1. Vaginal bleeding should cease in about six weeks

2. Increase participation in self-care activities gradually for two months

3. Report any missed period immediately to your physician

4. Use a barrier method of contraception for three months

26. The registered nurse is preparing to delegate nursing tasks on a women's health unit. Which of the following tasks should the nurse delegate to a licensed practical nurse?

1. Conduct a health history on a woman admitted with gonorrhea

2. Perform a physical examination on a young woman admitted with amenorrhea

3. Monitor the laboratory tests of a woman admitted to a women's health unit

4. Administer the analgesic drug before a cystocele repair

ANSWERS AND RATIONALES

1. 4. During a laparoscopy, carbon dioxide is injected into the abdomen to assist in visualizing the organs. The carbon dioxide remains in the body and moves up to the shoulder area in 24 hours, causing mild discomfort. The position for the procedure would not cause shoulder pain. Anxiety and muscle tension would not normally cause postprocedure shoulder pain. The shoulder pain is not referred pain related to the procedure.
NP = An
CN = Ph/7
CL = An
SA = 3

2. 2. If a client douches within two hours of a cervical culture, the results will be inaccurate, especially in terms of number of organisms present. Cultures can be taken at any time during the menstrual cycle and are not affected by sexual intercourse. Cervical and endometrial biopsies should not be done if a client is pregnant, but a cervical culture can be obtained and the results are not affected by pregnancy.
NP = As
CN = Ph/7
CL = Ap
SA = 3

3. 1. In the beginning stage of menopause, the woman experiences vaginal inelasticity and dryness, due to the declining levels of estrogen. Women entering menopause will begin to gain weight and their skin will become dry. As women start through menopause, they will have irregular menses for a period of time before they have amenorrhea.
NP = As
CN = Ph/8
CL = Ap
SA = 3

4. 3. The best way to prevent osteoporosis is a regular exercise program that includes weight bearing. Vitamins B_6 and E supplements are helpful in alleviating some of the clinical manifestations of menopause, but have no effect on osteoporosis. Immobility or lack of exercise with sedate hobbies will contribute to the development of osteoporosis. Estrogen, not progesterone, has a major effect on preventing loss of bone mass.
NP = Pl
CN = Ph/7
CL = Ap
SA = 3

5. 1. A lack of body fat and caloric intake affect hormonal function and are often the cause of secondary amenorrhea in thin, young athletes. Muscle tone does not affect hormone levels, nor does exercise postpone physical and physiological maturation. Exercise in any form will burn fat and thus contributes to the state of amenorrhea.
NP = An
CN = Ph/8
CL = An
SA = 3

6. 4. The pain of dysmenorrhea can generally be decreased by physical exercise, which provides neurophysiologic relief. Hot tub baths are recommended, but hot showers would not provide sufficient heat to the abdomen to provide relief. Increased salt and fluid intake would add to the existing bloating and retention of fluid, which would increase discomfort. The drug treatment of choice is use of prostaglandin inhibitors, not muscle relaxants.
NP = Im
CN = Ph/8
CL = Ap
SA = 3

7. 2, 3, 5. Raw parsley, celery, and asparagus are natural diuretics and are recommended for clients with premenstrual syndrome to reduce bloating

and edema. Cantaloupe, applesauce, and broccoli are all foods high in water content; they promote bloating and edema and are to be avoided.
NP = Im
CN = He/3
CL = Ap
SA = 3

8. 3. Menorrhagia is defined as prolonged or excessive vaginal bleeding with menses. Vaginal bleeding between menstrual periods is metrorrhagia. Pain with sexual intercourse is dyspareunia. Pain with the beginning of menstruation is dysmenorrhea.
NP = As
CN = Ph/8
CL = Ap
SA = 3

9. 2. One of the most important goals for a client with a rectovaginal fistula is the prevention of infection. *E. coli* in the rectum easily gains entrance to the vagina. Clients with a rectovaginal fistula do not have difficulty with physical mobility, and they do not have a change in body image often found with the loss of a body part. Clients with a rectovaginal fistula have perineal discomfort and irritation from the presence of stool in the vagina.
NP = Pl
CN = Ph/8
CL = An
SA = 3

10. 1. The client with a rectovaginal fistula needs to use measures that will prevent pressure at the site of the fistula. One of the measures is to increase fluid intake to prevent constipation and the resultant straining to have a bowel movement. The client should eat a low-residue diet. Paregoric is prescribed to inhibit bowel action, which would be contraindicated for this client. A vaginal tampon is also contraindicated, as it puts pressure on the area as it expands while absorbing the discharge.
NP = An
CN = Ph/7
CL = An
SA = 3

11. Vinegar. Vinegar is often used as an inexpensive solution for a deodorizing douche. A cleansing douche would use tap water or normal saline. Betadine is used as an antiseptic douching solution for preparing clients for vaginal surgery.
NP = Im
CN = He/3
CL = Ap
SA = 3

12. 1. A cystocele is a herniation of the bladder into the vagina. As a result of the herniation, the client experiences stress incontinence when laughing, walking, or lifting. The herniation does not cause any surface bleeding. Constipation and hemorrhoids are present with a rectocele.
NP = Ev
CN = Ph/8
CL = An
SA = 3

13. 4. One of the most important goals in the care of the client with a cystocele repair is prevention of infection, which would be detected with a change in vital signs. Postoperatively, clients should move all extremities in bed and ambulate as soon as possible to prevent thrombophlebitis. Urinary output should be monitored at least every four hours to ensure that no more than 100 ml of urine remains in the bladder at any one time. Clients with a cystocele repair do not have vaginal bleeding.
NP = As
CN = Ph/7
CL = Ap
SA = 3

14. 2. Kegel exercises reduce the symptoms of stress and urge incontinence. The exercises tighten and relax the muscles of the pelvic floor, but do not contract the muscles of abdomen or tighten pelvic organs. Kegel exercises do not alleviate pelvic pain.
NP = An
CN = He/3
CL = An
SA = 3

15. 3. The surgical procedure of an anterior and posterior colporrhaphy repairs the vaginal wall anteriorly and posteriorly to correct a cystocele and rectocele. Vaginal bleeding is not present unless there has been injury to the uterus. The client would normally have some pelvic discomfort. Since cathartics and enemas are prescribed preoperatively, it would be normal for the client not to have a bowel movement 48 hours postoperatively. This type of surgery is done vaginally or by laparoscopy; thus, there is no abdominal incision.
NP = Ev
CN = Ph/7
CL = An
SA = 3

16. **Prolapsed uterus.** A pessary is used to keep a prolapsed uterus in position when surgical repair is not an option. A pessary would not be used for a cystocele, uterine fibroids, or a bladder fistula.
    NP = Im
    CN = Ph/8
    CL = An
    SA = 3

17. 1. Frequent douching decreases the quantity of normal bacterial flora in the vagina and makes one more at risk for developing an infection. If performed properly, douching does not cause trauma to the vagina. Douching in and by itself does not alter sexual functioning or cause urge incontinence.
    NP = An
    CN = Ph/7
    CL = An
    SA = 3

18. 2'. The vaginal discharge in candidiasis is watery or thick with cottage cheese–like particles. A thick yellow purulent discharge is present in clients with chlamydia and gonorrhea. Clients with bacterial vaginosis have a gray discharge with a fishlike odor. Clients with trichomoniasis have a thin, yellow-brown, malodorous discharge.
    NP = As
    CN = Ph/8
    CL = Ap
    SA = 3

19. 2, 5, 6. Clients with acute pelvic inflammatory disease (PID) should be on bed rest in a semi-Fowler's position to facilitate dependent drainage and prevent abscess formation. Antibiotics are prescribed and safe sex practices are taught. Heat should be applied to the abdomen to increase circulation and promote comfort. Douching would be contraindicated in the acute phase. The client with PID has a purulent vaginal discharge, not blood.
    NP = Pl
    CN = Ph/7
    CL = Ap
    SA = 3

20. 2. Clinical manifestations of toxic shock become life threatening and may include loss of consciousness. The client with toxic shock syndrome initially has clinical manifestations of sudden high fever over 38.9°C, or 102°F, muscle pain, and hypotension.
    NP = An
    CN = Ph/7

CL = An
SA = 3

21. 1, 2, 6. Clients with uterine fibroids have excessive bleeding (menorrhagia) with their periods, low abdominal pressure, backache, and constipation. They do not have spotting between periods or pain with intercourse (dyspareunia).
NP = Ev
CN = Ph/7
CL = Ap
SA = 3

22. 3. Several episodes of vomiting could indicate the postoperative complication of a paralytic ileus. Faint bowel sounds, serosanguineous drainage in the suction apparatus at the surgical site, and vaginal bleeding are all normal assessments in the postoperative period.
NP = An
CN = Ph/7
CL = An
SA = 3

23. 2. Endometriosis occurs when endometrial cells are seeded outside the uterus and bleed into surrounding areas when stimulated by ovarian hormones. Pregnancy will create an anovulatory state, which will prevent the endometrial cells from responding to the ovarian hormones. The endometrial cells are seeded outside the uterus so controlling uterine bleeding will have little or no effect on relieving the clinical manifestations. Endometriosis is a chronic condition that continues until a woman reaches menopause. Exercise, nutrition, and rest are all important measures to help with pain control, but will not alleviate the clinical manifestations entirely.
NP = Pl
CN = He/3
CL = Ap
SA = 3

24. 1. The client with an ectopic pregnancy has a fertilized ovum implanted outside the uterus, most commonly in the fallopian tube. As the ovum grows it eventually ruptures the fallopian tube, resulting in shock. The client would be bleeding vaginally rather than having a mucus vaginal discharge. Difficulty in voiding occurs mainly when the uterus is enlarged. When the fallopian tube ruptures, the client experiences severe pain.
NP = Ev
CN = Ph/8
CL = Ap
SA = 3

25. 3. A client who had an ectopic pregnancy is at risk for another ectopic pregnancy, so any missed period should be evaluated by a physician. After treatment for an ectopic pregnancy, whether medically or surgically, the vaginal bleeding should cease within two to three weeks. Recovery from treatment should normally not require significant adjustments to self-care activities beyond six weeks. Once the pregnancy is terminated, the client can resume normal sexual activity with or without contraception after six weeks.
NP = Pl
CN = Ph/7
CL = Ap
SA = 3

26. 4. A licensed practical nurse may administer an analgesic drug before surgery. Conducting a health history, performing a physical examination, and monitoring laboratory tests are tasks that should be performed by a registered nurse.
NP = Pl
CN = Sa/1
CL = An
SA = 8